RETIN-A
AND OTHER
YOUTH MIRACLES

Joseph P. Bark, M.D.

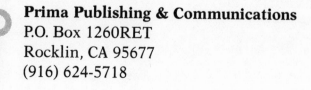

Prima Publishing & Communications
P.O. Box 1260RET
Rocklin, CA 95677
(916) 624-5718

Copy Editing by Anne Montague
Typography by Graphic Typesetting Service
Production by Robin Lockwood, Bookman Productions
Jacket Design by The Dunlavey Studio

Prima Publishing & Communications
Rocklin, CA

Library of Congress Cataloging-in-Publication Data

Bark, Joseph P.
  Retin-A and other youth miracles.

  Bibliography: p.
  Includes index.
  1. Tretinoin.   2. Skin—Aging—Prevention.
I. Title.
RL120.R48B37 1989   615′.778   89-3714
ISBN 0-914629-89-1

---

89 90 91 92 RRD 10 9 8 7 6 5 4 3 2 1

Printed in the United States of America

For Lin

A haven
A softness
A beauty
A light
A wellspring
An understanding
That inspires me
To seek these things for others . . .

Acknowledgments

As much as we may think that an idea belongs to one person and that one person alone, it does so only rarely. I have had vast amounts of assistance from my fellow dermatologists and the researchers who have so generously given of their time in uncovering the facts behind the wondrous drug Retin-A and all the procedures and techniques mentioned in this book.

Chief among those I must thank is Dr. Albert Kligman, whose position as pre-eminent researcher in the field of dermatology, and impassioned pleas for the humanization of medicine, have inspired every doctor and researcher to reach farther till it hurts for the very excellence he has mastered in his extraordinary career. He has always had the courage to stand up, head and shoulders above the rest, and be heard as a voice for the patient. Dr. Kligman believes in fighting what he calls "geronotphobia," the fear of aging, and I hope we dermatologists always have him by our side to guide us in our quest for a more comfortable life for our patients. His detailed review of this manuscript is greatly appreciated.

Thanks go to Dr. David Duffy, who not only hand-taught me a fine skill to serve patients for a lifetime but imparted a sensitivity for some of the problems and concerns of patients desiring cosmetic dermatological treatment. His insistence on excellence is a beacon in the darkness toward which all doctors must strive.

Dr. Arnold Fox, famed author and internist, gave me crucial assistance in planning chapters of this book and was kind enough to allow me to share this philosophy of aging in Chapter 16. Dr. Fox was the person who, years ago at the first AMA Health Reporting Conference, encouraged me to attempt a book project as a method for teaching more people the vital facts about dermatology. He shares my view that medicine should not be secretive, hidden information to be understood only by physicians. He, more than any doctor, knows the deep and abiding value of the "physician within us all."

My heartfelt thanks go to Dr. Paula Moynahan, who gave of her time in reviewing the information concerning plastic surgery. Her landmark text for laymen, *Cosmetic Surgery for Women*, is *the* guide for women *and* men to the difficult world of cosmetic surgery.

To Peggy Richards, who has kept me on track through a busy practice for 10 years, two books, media tours and lectures, travels, trips, trials, and tribulations, I give my sincere appreciation. She has offered many helpful hints on the organization of this book and has scanned it for its ability to impart information to the layman in words that are understandable.

I thank Debbie Mason Yates, who had to learn a whole new word processing system to help me through the morass of manuscript revisions. And moreover, her smiles and upbeat encouragement have seen all of us through this project with never a tense moment.

My thanks to Rhonda Greer, my chief clinical assistant, who has also reviewed parts of the manuscript. Her thoughtful maturity and calm under fire have helped us all hit the mark in preparation of this book.

To my agent and close friend Jim Heacock, for his understanding and enthusiasm for this project and my first book, *Skin Secrets*. His energy bubbles through two thousand miles of phone line, as he calls to tell me that "good news should always travel fast!" He is untiring in his pursuit of an audience for medical information that concerns us all. An outstanding and capable gentleman.

What a sincere pleasure it is to be able to thank an editor for all he has done with this manuscript. Ben Dominitz, my editor and publisher, is a superior fellow, who really took an interest in the Retin-A project. He's a virtual whirlwind of constructive ideas, and it's refreshing to work with one who cares for the work.

I thank Dr. Martin Luftman, plastic surgeon, and Dr. Emanuel Marritt, master of the hair transplant, for their valuable assistance in preparing the chapters on liposuction and hair, respectively. They are educators as well as physicians, who represent the epitome of our ideal of providing ethical information to the public.

To Tom Martin, Ortho Pharmaceutical representative, whose constant willingness to obtain the latest Retin-A information helped the progress of this book. If it's up to date, Mr. Martin is partially responsible. Hats off to this fine and ethical representative.

As in my last book, I am grateful to my friends and family who have had to share me with my laptop and this manuscript over the last 14 months.

Lastly, I would like to express my appreciation to all my radiaging patients who have been a part of my own experience in using Retin-A over the years. They have been a patient lot, as we gathered experiences together about the many applications of Retin-A.

Contents

Foreword

Most doctors can barely write a legible prescription. Very few can write clearly enough to communicate medical information that is understandable and accurate.

Communication skills are not taught in medical school. Doctors are either talking over the heads of patients, or talking down to them. Instead of receiving good medical counseling, the patient becomes confused and the therapeutic outcome is diminished.

Dr. Bark is a dramatic exception to jargon-spouting doctors. He is a no-nonsense physician who presents his material in an interesting and lucid way. Even more important, his medical teachings are sound and effective.

Dr. Bark is altogether unpretentious and personal in telling you what to do and what not to do. He knows a lot about skin, and a lot more about people.

Many years ago we first found Retin-A to be effective against common acne. I've always had an intense interest in this disease which virtually cripples so many teens and adults, and I reasoned that such a drug would really help. It did so very effectively. We watched cases of acne clear for years, while the patients described how much better their skin felt, but we should have been smarter. We should have *listened* to patients, as Dr. Bark obviously has. It took us years to see that Retin-A actually *does* improve the skin's texture, smooth minor lines, and correct some of the pigmentation and premalignancies of aging. But those realizations and others cited here by Dr. Bark came slowly. We thought it natural that patients would look better and feel better when their acne conditions improved. But they were telling us *more* than that. They were telling us that their skin had made a quantum leap toward feeling younger and smoother. Had *we* listened to *our* patients earlier, we might have discovered that photoaging is effectively reversed by this drug years before we did.

It was thrilling to be a part of the Retin-A story. And as the full potential of this drug is now being realized, it's gratifying to realize how many patients will be helped by it. I believe in Dr. Bark's "win-win" philosophy—the patient wins when the wrinkles subside on Retin-A, and the doctor wins when aging and sun damage are reversed.

Dr. Bark and I believe in direct and open communication with patients. Proper communication with your dermatologist is vital to the proper use of Retin-A. I'm not stumping for patients for dermatologists—God knows they have enough to do—but this new use of Retin-A needs to be supervised by the person who has experience with this drug, its minor complications, and all the ancillary hints and tips Dr. Bark talks about in *Retin-A and Other Youth Miracles*. This book can serve as your guidebook to using Retin-A for photoaging. Read the scientific facts about this drug, and see what it does and how it works. Study Dr. Bark's enlightened chapter on "The Day-to-Day Use of Retin-A," and you'll *know* the proper methods of application and hundreds of other facts that no other dermatologist has written down in this way for patients. In short, if you're going to use the *drug*, you'd be wise to read this *book* as a road map for Retin-A users.

The time has finally arrived that patients no longer submit meekly to doctors. They want to know the whys and wherefores of their treatments. The best patient is an informed one. Dr. Bark tells you virtually everything you need to know to get the most from your skin care program. This book will be extremely helpful to *anyone* interested in improving his or her looks as the years pass. Retin-A *is* a wonderful medicine for use in photoaging. I agree with Dr. Bark and his enthusiasm for this drug, and I'm happy I could be a small part in this saga of Retin-A.

Albert M. Kligman, MD, PhD
Department of Dermatology
University of Pennsylvania
School of Medicine
Philadelphia, PA 19104

Before You Read Anything Else: A Few Cautions on the Use of This Book

Several points need to be emphasized before you begin this book:

1. No amount of written advice can substitute for your own dermatologist's care—not this book, nor *any* book. Books can just tell you what medicines are available and how to use them effectively. But your own dermatologist must be your final guide. Furthermore, if you choose to use a non–skin specialist to safeguard the health of your body's largest, most visible organ, then you're not as smart as you appeared to be when you bought this book.

2. Retin-A has not yet been approved by the Food and Drug Administration (FDA) for use in reversing wrinkles, sun damage, blotches, premalignancies, or photoaging (what I like to call "radiaging"). Retin-A was originally developed as an anti-acne medication. You would be using this medicine (or some others I mention herein) for a non-approved indication. However, once a drug is approved for *any* indication, there is ample precedent for its use in other skin conditions. This is a judgment that has been the privilege of the *doctor*, not the bureaucrat. Be aware that "nonapproved" does *not* mean "ineffective." If such uses were against the law, every dermatologist would have spent significant time and trouble reaching through bars

1

to treat his or her patients. Even the officials of the FDA call this "accepted medical practice."

Be aware that on July 6, 1988, the FDA *did* issue a warning that the drug was as yet unapproved for photoaging, and, thankfully, that officials would be cracking down on those who claim to be selling Retin-A but are not. Many bogus vitamin A formulations have hit the market. Retin-A is available only on a doctor's prescription from the Ortho Pharmaceutical Corporation, a division of Johnson & Johnson, and is available in *no other forms, cosmetics, or creams*. The old saw still applies: *Let the buyer beware!* Similar-sounding names are a tipoff to a counterfeit.

3. This book is written so *you* can understand it. You may take it to your dermatologist to ask for help in designing a skin care program especially for your individual skin. Certain modifications are necessary to tailor any medical program to the individual patient's needs and skin type. Your dermatologist will appreciate your interest and knowledge of the subject, and your preparation, so take this book with you to his or her office and ask for advice!

The preceding sentence is the last time in this book where "his or her" will be used. I polled 100 of my private patients at random, and 97 said they preferred the pronoun *his* over the boring, clumsy, and overworked construction. I would have been just as willing to use *her*, but my survey showed people clearly preferred the one I shall use throughout this book. No offense is intended by this usage.

4. I will be happy to answer your questions, but only if you send along a self-addressed, stamped, business-size envelope with your query. Otherwise they go into that great all-American institution, the wastebasket. Here's my address:

RETIN-A
Box 22253
Lexington, KY 40522

Introduction

Beauty has always been extremely important.
All cultures have rewarded and praised beauty.
The ancient Egyptians, thousands of years
before Cleopatra, used cosmetics to enhance
their natural beauty. Appearance is even more
important today. Teachers favor pretty
children. Beautiful people get the dates and the
mates. Good-looking job applicants win out
over uglier prospects. Even we medical people
prefer to treat attractive patients rather than
those with repugnant disease. Good-looking
people feel better about themselves, and they
succeed more in life. So we shouldn't be
surprised that patients are willing to cooperate
for years with a treatment regimen that
promises them a better appearance.

—*Albert M. Kligman, MD, father of Retin-A*

When you reached for this book, you expressed a desire to stay young. When I wrote this book, I made a commitment to teach you how to do just that. When Dr. Albert Kligman, the father of Retin-A, says, "The object of aesthetic dermatology is to help you die young as *late* as possible," he means just that. While we have no "cure" for the aging process, we are all living longer, and in better health. It cannot be said too strongly that it truly *is* possible to look better (even *marvelous*) while the years march on. Someone said, "Aging is better than the alternative." Who

---

Youth Alert!

If you have the opportunity to guide or advise your kids on sports activities, try to get them excited about indoor sports, such as gymnastics, skating, dancing. To do so is to keep them away from the damaging rays of the sun during the period (before age 18) when they'll get 80% of the sun damage of their entire lives!

---

could disagree? But you don't need to *look* your age or to broadcast it to anyone.

Maintaining a youthful appearance is usually thought of as the prerogative of women, but Retin-A and many other new advances in dermatology and plastic surgery will change all that. Nobody, man or woman, need look his chronological age these days. Premature aging is often a result of cumulative environmental injury and is certainly avoidable. And if you follow my advice about sunscreens, your *kids* will probably look even better than *you* when they're your age.

My own lessons in photoaging started at a very young age. As a kid, I loved amusement parks. I especially loved to go with my family to the Cedar Point amusement park in northern Ohio. Luckily, my father always taught me to observe the finest details of life, and the amusement park was a wonderful place to practice his advice.

One day, while watching the barkers along the midway of the park, I saw a wrinkled old guy in a small booth shouting that he could tell anyone's age for a quarter; if

---

Youth Alert!

Laxity of the skin on the backs of the hands is one of the very earliest signs of radiaging!

---

he could not pinpoint it within three years, he would award his customer a huge stuffed animal. I was amazed at his success, which, over the summer approached 70%! The way I figured it, this guy should have taken his skills to the racetrack a long time ago. I decided to study his successes more intently.

As I watched, I could see the man step back and "size up" his mark, complimenting each on the difficulty in age-estimating "such a young-looking specimen." He certainly won a lot of friends that way, and some of them convinced *their* friends to come over to "play the game." The women would extend their hands when he offered his greeting, almost bowing while saying hello. Meanwhile, he gently pinched the skin on the back of the woman's hand.

It was not until many years later in my dermatology residency that I discovered he was using one of the most reliable dermatologic age predictors: the "pinch test." It's a simple test you can do to spot early skin radiaging in a very common site—on the backs of the hands. If you pinch up the skin there (try it on your own hand!), you can tell a person's approximate age by how fast the skin snaps back. Fast is young, slow is old, and of course there are all stages of aging in between. (This is such an accurate predictor of skin aging that researchers have developed a machine to do it more accurately! The instrument is called a "twistometer." The pinch test was also used after the atomic bombs were dropped on Japan, to evaluate the skin of survivors years later.)

The midwayman I watched that summer had really become quite a skin specialist, having pinched enough hands to know when he was holding one of a 30-, 40-, or 50-year-old! Of course, I saw him look intently at some pretty severe facial wrinkles, drooping eyelids, lengthening noses and age spots, too, so he knew a lot more than the average customer would realize about aging. He was indeed a keen observer.

Our midwayman could rarely guess the correct age of a black woman. "Fifty-six!" he'd say, before checking the

===== *Youth Alert!* =====

Why does a black woman's skin appear to age more slowly than that of a Caucasian? The black's built-in sunscreen (melanin pigment) stops most of the damage from sun exposure. That's just one more indication that wrinkles are largely sun-induced.

driver's license of a 65-year-old, or "Forty-five!" for a 58-year-old. In fact, I perceived that he was almost angry when a black woman paid for his "guess." He knew he'd almost certainly lose one of his big prizes if he accepted her challenge. Why did he have so much trouble predicting the age of black skin? Because the high sun protection afforded by its melanin pigment had prevented radiaging.

Years later, I cringed when I watched the way the makeup artists incorrectly aged Cicely Tyson in *The Autobiography of Miss Jane Pittman*, the wonderful TV miniseries about an aging black woman's quest for equality. They created wrinkles too early to indicate that she had aged. Excessive sun exposure can damage black skin too, but much later. Melanin is less effective in blocking the longer ultraviolet rays (called UVA), which are more abundant in sunlight and are present the year round. So even blacks have to heed the sun warnings given by dermatologists. (Caucasian women should take a lesson in wrinkle prevention from the skin of black women: Protect yourself from the sun and avoid all the ugly signs of radiaging.)

At the Jefferson Medical College "Biology of Aging Skin" conference in May 1988, Dr. Kligman showed photographs of a 50-year-old woman whose face had so many wrinkles it looked like lizard skin. She had become addicted to the sun at an early age, and her skin had been irrevocably destroyed by it by the age of 30! Then he showed a slide of an Asian gentleman who looked, I'd say, in his early to middle 50s—it was hard to tell, he had so little wrinkling. After letting us guess a few seconds, Dr. Kligman told us the man was actually *90* years old! But he had virtually *never* received any sun damage, being a contemplative religious monk who had never gone outdoors.

So while actual chronological aging ("intrinsic" aging) proceeds unabated as yet by medical science, we really do know some marvelous ways to stave off the sun-induced *appearance* of aging (radiaging), and at last to actually *reverse* some of its effects. That's what this book is all about—keeping the same glow of youth in and on your skin that is in your mind and in your heart. I guarantee that you'll look younger for the rest of your years if you follow this program diligently.

Of course, the object is not to make everyone look like a 20-year-old—we all know that is just not possible with today's science and technology. But it *is* possible to have a more *youthful* look for whatever age we are. Aging *can*, indeed, be done gracefully, and for each age, we all know someone who looks great for his age, and someone else who looks like the proverbial horse that's been "rode hard and put up wet"! The object, then, is to be of the first group—the group that looks the best for each and every age. As a matter of fact, protected, unexposed skin shows only very slight changes until after age 60. So, much can be done! Now here's a brief overview of what you'll find in subsequent pages.

We'll review the newest protective measures that can stop sun damage literally in its tracks, including the newest and most effective sunscreens, which can protect even the lightest, most sun-sensitive skin around.

You will learn all about the drug Retin-A. I'll discuss the history of that compound and some of its relatives and teach you the proper ways to use it to reverse radiaging. We'll discuss the newest and most photoprotective cosmetics as an adjunct to beauty and health.

Another chapter will introduce you to the world of beautiful legs. Or legs that are *again* beautiful, through what can only be described as a dermatologic art form, injection of unsightly veins. You'll hardly believe the success of this marvelous and safe procedure, which I had the privilege of learning from the master of the art, Dr. David Duffy of Torrance, California. In this chapter, you'll learn about the solutions used for the vein injections, the success rate, treatment regimen, and complications of treating large and small leg veins.

I'll discuss hair loss, new advances in the use of minoxidil for regrowth of lost hair, and other ways to correct the apparent signs of aging with "youth surgery"—the magic nips and tucks used by the dermatologic and plastic surgeons to hide the years.

You'll learn some important tips about injectable collagen, silicone, and a new material, Fibrel, as well as autologous fat transplants and some advanced techniques for redistributing and removing excess body fat.

One chapter deals with the many advances in basic science that are being made to try to slow down the actual aging process. I will present exciting facts about vitamins, beta carotene, newer compounds intended to retard the process, and exercise as a means to maintaining good skin tone.

If you read this book seriously, especially in regard to the use of Retin-A, you may indeed be able to drop years from your appearance. And when you *look* better, you'll *feel* better too. The plastic surgeons call that having a "good body image." And when you feel better, your whole life will improve. As Maria, a Retin-A patient of mine, says, "Retin-A's not perfect—I guess nothing really is. It irritates sometimes, and it's a bother to put it on all the time. But my skin looks smoother and feels tighter and less wrinkled now, and that's what really matters to me. I wouldn't give up that medicine for *anything*!" It's my fervent hope that some of the information you find here will help you look and feel better, and *younger*, just like Maria. After all, that's everybody's quest!

Throughout this book, I've highlighted what I call "*Youth Alerts!*" These are designed to make it easier for you to skim through the text to find the highlights of current concern. But don't try to use just them for customizing your own program. As I've said, that requires the help of your dermatologist, and the reading and study of every word in the program outline provided here.

Now, go find a nice chair somewhere, and get ready to learn about good skin care and staying young. And good luck!

Part 1

The Retin-A Story

1

Retin-A: What's Behind the Furor?

Every Caucasian woman past age 15 has serious structural changes in her facial skin.
—*Albert M. Kligman, MD*

No one who was ever concerned about his appearance will ever forget that night in January 1988 when the network TV newscasts all had headline stories like this:

"Scientists in today's *Journal of the American Medical Association* tell us that a drug used in acne treatment for some 15 years has now been found effective in actually *reversing* some of the signs of aging from the sun. This medicine, called Retin-A, has been found to erase wrinkles in test subjects, and is now under wider trial in the U.S. to obtain FDA approval for such use."

That news about Retin-A (also called vitamin A acid, retinoic acid, or tretinoin [tret-in-OH-in]) amply demonstrated that it is a most remarkable agent. For the next couple of weeks, follow-up stories appeared in the *Washington Post, USA Today*, the *Wall Street Journal*, and almost every local newspaper in America about the "Fountain of Youth" cream. I myself gave over 30 interviews about Retin-A in the first week following the announcement! No one had to be convinced this was major news, and was likely to remain major news for some time. Even the comics picked up the story.

13

And the story was so big that it even spilled over our borders. On January 31, 1988, the Associated Press reported that a little town just over the U.S.-Mexico border had been inundated with requests for the drug, a nonprescription item in that country. Pharmacists in Matamoros, Mexico, were selling every tube of the cream they could get their hands on, at the usual Mexican price of $1.20 for 10 grams (the usual price in the States was about $18.95 for a 20-gram tube). The article quoted U.S. Customs officials as saying they would confiscate any of the cream coming into this country unless the person had a valid U.S. prescription for it.

But it was apparently a gamble many were, and still are, willing to take. The problem with such purchases, aside from not having the correct instructions for use of the substance, is that people were buying all the forms, including the potent gels and liquid form. Unhappily, it was not long till we in the United States started seeing the complications of such "self- prescribing." Retin-A is a potent drug that cannot be used carelessly or casually.

On February 12, 1988, the *Wall Street Journal* published a front-page piece on Retin-A that reported some really harsh complaints about the new "Retin-A-mania" from some pharmacy school representatives. Jere Goyan, dean of the school of pharmacy at the University of Southern California, said about the possible side effects: "It can be frightening. How would you feel if you woke up and your eyes were swelled shut?"

Most dermatologists thought of these as scare tactics, if not frankly hysterical. I especially liked the comment in *Dermatology Times*, March 1988, by Dr. John J. Vorhees, one of the principal investigators in the controlled study of Retin-A reported in the *Journal of the American Medical Association*. "Detractors of this drug are just that: detractors." His point was that dermatologists whose patients use this potent drug are well aware of the side effects of Retin-A.

Beware of the "Bait-and-Switch"!

The Retin-A phenomenon hit this country while I was still touring the talk show circuit for my previous book, *Skin Secrets*. Almost overnight, I witnessed the spawning of entire Retin-A *clinics*, occasionally sponsored by plastic surgeons and other ambitious nondermatologists who saw an opportunity to enhance their surgery-oriented practices. They were anxious to jump into the Retin-A waters— where they could find a ready source of aging patients who could be sold a lot of surgical operations along with a little Retin-A.

In my years in medicine, I had never witnessed anything or any movement so momentous. Cosmetic companies virtually stopped their production lines to toss in a little fake Retin-A, usually useless forms of vitamin A known for years to do nothing to human skin except maybe grease it up a little. In my opinion, these "me too" products should have been named "Avarice Cream" and "Greed Lotion"! These gimmicks were never meant to separate you from your wrinkles—just from your money!

It was troubling to us dermatologists when we saw patients falling for the lies promulgated by the various cosmetic companies. I occasionally visit cosmetic counters in strange cities just to see what lines of malarkey the salespersons are dealing out to the age-conscious public. Often I hear words like, "Oh, don't listen to that Retin-A stuff—that stuff will rip your face off, and doesn't do you nearly as much good as our Impassioned Zitella Skin Refluxing System! Why, you use our elegant products and you'll start wanting to bathe in a bassinet and cruise toy stores in just four short weeks!" Garbage, pure and simple.

But behind the hype there *was* a lot of legitimate research into the real product, Retin-A. The solid scientific work was getting lost in all the hullaballoo over this drug's apparent effectiveness in reducing and reversing wrinkles. Oh, reversing wrinkles and the *look* of aging is important, all right, and is the main thrust of this book. But there's a wealth of additional information about its effects on all the various skin cells and layers that you also need to understand in order to use the medicine intelligently.

Common Objections to Using Retin-A

First, let's address some of the most common questions about Retin-A and some of the fears that rightfully accompany any new use for a potent drug such as this.

What about the person who is a "naturalist"—someone who wants everything he applies to his skin or takes internally to be "natural" or "of nature"? Should such a person consider Retin-A? *Naturally*! What could be more natural than vitamin A? It's the quintessential natural substance—we can't live without it; that's why it's called a "vitamin," which came from "vital amine."

Shouldn't we just let nature take its course? Isn't it unnatural, by definition, to be fiddling around with the aging process? (This argument is often proffered by those who think that if God had meant man to fly, He'd have given him wings.) Of course not. Wrinkles are not natural—they're just a product of our times, and certainly a new product of new times, at that. As you'll see in subsequent chapters, dermatologists look back longingly at the bonnet generations of times past.

Doesn't Retin-A *cause* cancers? How about the warnings on the package insert, that persons using this drug should assiduously avoid sunlight? Don't even a lot of *pharmacists* tell their clients that? There is *no* human experience that bears this out. In almost 20 years of experience with this drug, in fact, just the opposite is true: the drug Retin-A *protects* against skin cancers as do all the retinoids, or vitamin A derivatives. And use of Retin-A is becoming *more* important to all of us every single day, as our thin protective layer of ozone wears out under the onslaught of modern industry and chemicals.

Should we wait until something better comes along? After all, aren't there hundreds of similar compounds under development right now, which will do the job of reversing radiaging and wrinkles without all the irritation and the dangers of Retin-A? Hey, I'd be a fool to argue with the fact that there will always be something better to come along. Our modern age (which, by the way, has gone in my lifetime from the Air Age to the Jet Age to the Space Age and who knows what next) will always produce a better product. That's just a fact that defines the nature of progress. But to delay for who-knows-how-many-years the fine effects that can be achieved with Retin-A is just cheating yourself.

In fact, this question reminds me of a close friend of mine (also a doctor) who resisted for years buying a computer for his growing medical practice. He waited and waited, maintaining that "the best was yet to come" in hardware and software for his office, until his patient accounts were hopelessly muddled and his accountant finally stepped in and twisted his arm. Now he's in seventh heaven with his new setup, and his practice is thriving. Of *course* there is some new and better system somewhere now, but he has one that is perfectly adequate for him, just as, comparatively, Retin-A can be perfectly adequate for you for many years.

I told much the same thing to one "friend" with whom I discussed the idea of doing this book, while it was still a twinkle in my eye. "Joe," said the head-shaking friend, "sure, it's Retin-A this year, but it'll be Retin-*B* next year, and nobody will give a hoot about the current drug! Your book will be passé before it gets to the stores!" Maybe there *will* be new drugs on the distant horizon, but by George, I'm not going to withhold the facts about using Retin-A while people continue to expose themselves to the aging effects of the sun and tanning booths. We have it in our power to do something *now* about the way our skins

=== *Youth Alert!* ===

The morning after the announcements about wrinkle correction with Retin-A were made, we dermatologists dubbed it, "the vanishing cream," because it was snatched off the pharmacy shelves all over the nation in just a matter of hours by patients hungry for its effects!

are aging, and about how we look as the years pass. And I, for one, think this opportunity must be taken.

Oh, this book's not a real Fountain of Youth. Retin-A will help your skin look better, and it will prevent some of the skin cancers that we see all too often these days, but it *is* a start toward a better and more comfortable aging process. And Retin-A is a very important part of that process—to whose secrets more and more vital keys are being discovered almost daily.

What *Is* Retin-A?

In 1969, Dr. Albert Kligman discovered a direct vitamin A derivative and its most active metabolite (breakdown product), vitamin A acid, to be very effective in topical form in the treatment of acne. This compound loosened the attachments between epidermal cells, a significant advance in the treatment of acne, because blackheads and whiteheads form because epidermal cells stick together to plug up the follicular openings. These plugs (comedones) could then rupture and dump their contents into the skin, producing pustules and pimples. If these plugs were loosened with Retin-A, the theory went, acne could be alleviated in many, many victims. The fact is that the plugs cannot form on Retin-A therapy, so the primary lesions of acne are prevented. Already existing comedones loosen and fall out, forestalling pimples.

Over the next few years, Retin-A was proved to be one of the best drugs we had for most types of acne; the best "responders" were those patients with comedonal (blackhead and whitehead) acne, but almost every type of acne responded to some degree. To this day, Retin-A is the most frequently prescribed dermatological medicine, and it was even before the famous studies of Kligman and Vorhees regarding its use in radiaging, which have possibly doubled its sales.

In studies 30 years ago in the United States and Europe, Retin-A was shown to be helpful in some uncommon hereditary skin disorders. One of these conditions, called icthyosis (meaning "fish skin," because of the terrible skin scaling of these patients), was so dramatically helped that the patients who used the medicine were, for the first time, able to leave their houses without being shunned. This compound was subsequently used for a great variety of skin diseases (everything from psoriasis to the "mask of pregnancy," those brownish stains women sometimes develop on their faces after delivery or while on the pill), at least on a trial basis, and a large number of diseases have proven very responsive to it (see Appendix). In fact, some of these diseases had never been treatable previously, except with high-dose, toxic amounts of oral vitamin A that could not be used for extended periods.

After reading many of the studies involving these diseases and their successful treatment with Retin-A, I'm amazed that its only FDA-approved indication is for the treatment of acne. No doubt, when the data are submitted to the FDA, Retin-A will be approved for radiaging. In fact, Retin-A was even tried *orally*, long before its safer relatives, Accutane (1981) and Tegison (1986), were developed for acne and psoriasis, respectively. In the oral trials, Retin-A was effective but proved much too toxic.

Why Not Oral Vitamin A?

Since Retin-A is a vitamin A derivative, you may ask your-self, as many have, why oral vitamin A was not the best approach. After all, it would be simple to take a couple of pills a day to reverse the signs of aging and the other skin diseases for which Retin-A seems to be effective.

The vitamin retinol (vitamin A) is necessary to health in small amounts. It's obtained from many dietary sources such as green and yellow vegetables, and is stored in the liver. *Retinoids* are vitamin A–*like* compounds that are created in the research laboratory by modifying the basic vitamin A molecule and adding certain substances that change the chemical action of vitamin A.

In this way, thousands of truly different "designer drugs" can be created, each with different actions and toxicities, or poisonous properties. (That's a fact that all too few people really consider about the potent drugs many patients take these days. But toxic potential exists for almost *any* substance, including *water*, if used incor-rectly!) Remember, too, that the retinoids, including Retin-A, are being used not as vitamins but as drugs—not to maintain health, but to correct disease.

Scientists found out long ago about the severe toxicity that can occur with overdoses of dietary vitamin A. The classic example is the Arctic explorers who thought it was safe to eat the liver of polar bears. Eskimos were aware of the dangers of eating this part of the polar bear and had avoided it like the plague, but newly arrived explorers knew nothing of this. So the explorers ate the liver, a mis-take that caused acute poisoning from the massive amounts of vitamin A it contained (some 600,000 units per ounce—the daily requirement is only 5,000 units). The same symptoms of vitamin A toxicity happen when it's given in high dosage capsule form for severe skin diseases.

Chronic vitamin A toxicity from overdosage is not a pretty sight. The symptoms include dryness of the skin, headaches, chapped lips, bone and joint pain, hair loss, easy blistering of the skin in areas of trauma, elevation of cholesterol and triglycerides, severe irritation of the liver, and many other symptoms.

The clinical results in some rare skin diseases were good, however, despite these adverse side effects. For many, it was worth the risk. This prompted a search for a way to use vitamin A without taking it internally.

So vitamin A was tried topically (rubbed on) as early as 1932, but was completely ineffective when used in this way. Later, it was found that its chief metabolite, vitamin A acid, *was* effective topically.

Retin-A and Pregnancy

Internally administered retinoids—Accutane, the most potent acne drug, and Tegison, used in the treatment of psoriasis—can cause fetal malformations if taken by a pregnant woman. Tegison must never even be given to a woman of childbearing *potential*. In high doses, vitamin A itself can cause congenital malformations.

But in 1975, at the First World Congress on Topical Retinoic Acid, researchers agreed that topical vitamin A acid (Retin-A) was not harmful to fetuses. Retin-A was but slightly absorbed, and the concentrations used were low. Recently, applications to large body areas were found not to result in increased blood levels. The effects are purely local, at the site of application. Interestingly, the package insert *still* says that Retin-A is not for use in pregnancy, even though no birth defect problems have occurred in millions of pregnant young women who used Retin-A for acne.

Let me tell you what the drug's discoverer, and most experienced user, Dr. Albert M. Kligman, has to say about that matter. At the Biology of Human Skin Aging conference in the spring of 1988, he was asked whether we should use Retin-A in pregnant women. He bristled at the implication that Retin-A should be avoided in pregnancy. "We physicians," stormed Kligman, "have got to have the courage to do what we think is right for our patients. We have never heard of a problem in pregnancy due to this drug. It's high time that someone stand up and say that it is not going to cause a problem!"

On the other hand, when the same question was put to Dr. Vorhees, the investigator who published the January 1988 study on the efficacy of using Retin-A in reversing radiaging, he said, "No, I do *not* use it in pregnancy. Not that I feel there would ever be any problem with it. I do not. But in every hundred pregnancies, there are one or two congenital abnormalities, and I would not want to see Retin-A falsely incriminated in these cases." He thought it the better part of valor for the physician to refrain from using it in pregnancy.

My advice to you is this: If you are pregnant, consult with your obstetrician or family physician about using any drug.

Some Happy Acne Patients!

The acne patients using Retin-A reported to their doctors that they liked the "rosy glow" and other cosmetic effects the medicine produced. Dr. Kligman and his co-workers noted that some patients who were on topical Retin-A for several years seemed to be aging less rapidly. The rosy glow and skin tightness these patients reported were accompanied by a general lessening of wrinkles and a resolution of some of the signs of radiaging caused by the sun, as opposed to the "intrinsic" aging that happens chronologically to us all, sun-exposed or not. These observations made it worthwhile to study Retin-A as a possible adjunct to *correction* of radiaging. No one ever thought that possible, but when the studies that you'll read about in this book were done, there was indeed a noticeable reversal of radiaging.

Dermatologists heard from Dr. Kligman about the promising studies of Retin-A's use in radiaging as far back as 1986, and many of us have been using the drug for this purpose since that time. In my own office, I've used this medication with hundreds of patients, about 80%–90% of them women (I say this regretfully—many men who need care don't seek it), who have had almost every reported side effect and good effect from the medicine, some which had not previously been reported. In succeeding chapters, I'll tell you about my personal experiences.

Here's an interesting footnote to this brief history of Retin-A. Most of you probably figure that Dr. Kligman is the recipient of most of the profit associated with the sales of Retin-A (estimated in the *Wall Street Journal* article to top $60 million in 1988, as compared with $35 million in 1987). This is not so. He voluntarily relinquished his Retin-A patent rights to the Department of Dermatology at the University of Pennsylvania School of Medicine, which receives all the royalties.

We are now at a scientific threshold. It's a time of exciting discoveries that may change the way we live, and even allow us to shove some sand back up into the hourglass. Maybe, just maybe we're on the verge of extending our normal "three score and ten," by many, many more years, looking great all the while, with the help of astounding chemical advances like Retin- A. Maybe this book will be your personal beginning in that quest. What this book *can* do is let you look far younger than your years, and let you live those years more comfortably, with a better self-image. After all, most of us are taking better care of our bodies these days, and I think it's time we do everything we can to keep looking young and feeling young, while science studies ways to extend our life span.

2

Radiaging: Slow Death of All the Skin Under the Sun

If you want to have baby-ass skin when you're 90, lead a shady life!
—*Albert M. Kligman, MD*

A perfect covering formed of billions of cells has grown over us in the form of skin. And if you think of it, isn't it truly remarkable that, until middle and old age, almost everyone's skin fits him perfectly! Unfortunately, as in many recognized illnesses, the body starts out with tissues in wonderful arrangement, but they're destroyed progressively by the way we *use* them, or by what we *apply* to them, or by what *shines* on them.

In the Introduction I mentioned the pinch test, a sign that betrays the level of radiaging. If you haven't tried it on your own skin yet, you should to see what shape your own skin is in. Pinch up the skin on the back of one hand, release it, and watch how fast it returns. You say it doesn't exactly snap back, but more accurately could be described as an amazingly slow crawl back? That indicates that you already have significant *radiaging*, my favorite term for the *aging* process induced in all levels of the skin by the sun's *radi*ation.

========= *Youth Alert!* =========

The hands tell it all! If you really want to begin to appreciate how easy it is to predict age, look at the hands first, not the face. Many women protect their faces with cosmetics, which partially block the sun, but they do not take the same care with their hands. This is eminently evident when you start trying to estimate the age of others.

The properties of the skin that make it snap back in youth but not later on, after significant radiaging, are the subject of this chapter. And while some of the explanation of collagen and other chemicals and structures in the skin is somewhat technical, it's useful for those who really want to know how to take care of their skin.

It's my aim in this chapter to show you as exactly as possible how *structure* relates to *function* of the skin. If you can imagine your tiny collagen bundles breaking the next time you feel the warm, comfortable sun on your hands while at the beach, you may just think twice before soaking up those rays.

Just as in any other medical field, informed action is better than blind acceptance of a treatment program. When my editor asked me about the necessity to explain all this, I asked him whether he thought he'd get better service at the mechanic's if he was a mechanical wizard and let that be known, or if he walked in and said, "I've got no idea what's wrong with this car—just *fix* the thing, and send me the bill!"

Your Skin's Reaction to Sunlight

What happens in radiaging? What have all those tropical vacations and trips to the tanning salon done for you? To put it simply, the orderly architecture of the dermis and epidermis, the two top layers of the skin, is slowly and progressively annihilated by sunlight. Let me take you on a guided tour of normal skin and at the same time contrast this normal anatomy with the disastrous and widespread changes that occur in radiaging.

To take this tour, we'll start our descriptions of skin from the outside in. Think about your own skin as you go through the following sections, because you'll be able to spot your own signs of radiaging as you read each paragraph. I don't intend to scare you with all this, but often it's necessary to look very closely at the *problem* in order to understand the *solution*.

The Dead Skin Layer: Your Protective Envelope

The outermost skin layer is called the stratum corneum. Though dead, it is of immense value in protecting our skin's inner layers. Most people know it as the layer that creates, along with dissolved soap, the ring in the bathtub. But it does infinitely more than that! It's one of the true guardians of the skin, sloughing off constantly to cleanse it and to remove potentially harmful bacteria, and to adjust the acidity of its surface to insure that only the "right" bacteria grow.

Most important, this dead layer is relatively impermeable, so that noxious chemicals find it almost impossible to penetrate into the deeper layers, and it renews *itself* daily and constantly, as long as it's needed. Quite simply put, life on land would be impossible without it. The outer layer is the Saran Wrap in which we are all encased—a barrier against the entrance of harmful substances, and a buffer against sun and trauma. It also prevents us from drying out!

Chronic sun exposure causes the dead layer to thicken, become rougher, scalier, dryer, and less flexible. It can crack and even weep.

Think of this rough example: I once met a teenager in a diving class named Bobbi, who was what I call a "tanning freak." Although a Caucasian, she was a deep mahogany. Bobbi had terrific features—one of those kids who, if not so sun-damaged, could have stepped right into Eileen Ford's agency as a top fashion model. She signed in to my office one day for a minor skin problem, and asked how I thought she was doing with her skin. I really think she was quite proud of the way she looked. I hated to tell her about the sun damage she was courting, but someone had to.

"Bobbi, I've got some good news and some bad news for you," I said, trying to reassure her a little. "First the bad news—you've got quite a bit of sun damage and early wrinkling from your quest for the Great American Tan."

"But Dr. Bark!" she protested, "I always wear a sunscreen when I'm outside. Why do *I* have a problem?"

On further questioning I found out that she used only an SPF (sun protection factor) 4 sunscreen on her face, and a 2 on her body—if she felt really conscientious during a tanning session, that is. For real protection, SPF 15 and above is recommended. On most days, she'd just used some lotion designed to produce the darkest, deepest tan possible. It had no real sunscreen in it at all, just oils to *promote* tanning. They accomplish that nefarious purpose by making the dead layer of the skin more transparent. That's an invitation for the sun's rays to really nuke your skin! In other words, she was intensifying the damage.

"OK," she conceded, "please go ahead and give me the *good* news—I think I need it!"

"The good news is that it's not too late to restore the damage. Your skin is basically beautiful, and your facial symmetry is astounding. But we must act quickly to preserve and restore the texture of your skin."

I asked her to remove her cosmetics so that I could examine her facial skin more effectively. Under magnification, the incredible number of small sun wrinkles on her skin shocked me. All around her eye sockets were

---

Youth Alert!

A tanned look is not a healthy look! It's a leathery, thickened, awful look—we dermatologists know it from treating patients every day. Now even the modeling agencies are waking up to that fact.

---

hundreds of fine lines—called "crinkles" by some dermatologists—evidence that the sun had marched across this smooth, once youthful skin and was starting to leave its ugly aging tracks. The surface had completely lost its youthful smoothness, and the dead layer felt stiff, unbending, and rough—and all this in a 17-year-old!

Sun-Damaged Epidermis—A Dilapidated Brick Wall

The dead layer is made by the first living layer of the skin, the epidermis. It was here where beautiful Bobbi's skin showed the worst changes. I couldn't help thinking of one of the best analogies we dermatologists use to explain these changes: the old leather coat.

Have you ever seen an old piece of leather that has hung in a closet, or worse yet, out in the sun for several years? The leather gets so sun-worn that, on bending, it actually cracks! Human skin exposed to sun does much the same. No wonder many people itch after sun exposure!

During sun exposure, the epidermis also becomes much less protective. It allows irritants to enter more freely and becomes allergic to chemicals much more easily. We dermatologists see this in practice as a tendency toward dry, scaly skin that some patients are forever trying to repair with various moisturizers, lotions, and potions. How many middle-aged women with sun damage have a virtual cabinetful of moisturizers to soften their rough skin? Of course, not all dryness in middle or later age is attributable to sun changes in the dead layer, but much of it is.

The same sun that thickens the dead layer eventually causes drastic *thinning* of the first living layer, the epidermis. In fact, biopsy specimens show that this layer's thickness can go from a youthful *20* cells down to only 2 or 3 cells after chronic radiaging. If you could see it, you'd wonder how we could even survive with only a handful of thin, abnormal, sun-damaged epidermal cells to protect us. It's another tribute to the resiliency of the skin.

In practice, this thinning means a whole lot for the health and beauty of your skin. For one thing, thin skin bends much more easily, causing wrinkling that we'll talk about more in Chapter 3. Interestingly, the sun damage that thins out your skin actually perpetuates itself, because once thinned, your skin admits even *more* sunlight, causing even more thinning and wrinkling: a classic vicious circle!

And if that thinning weren't enough, more important changes have taken place during your years of tanning. The epidermis is normally a virtual model of organization. If you examined a bit of baby skin under a microscope, you'd see one of the most beautifully organized structures in creation. In fact, some investigators have equated the normal, undamaged epidermis to the arrangement of stones in a brick wall—neat, perfectly oriented stacks of cellular "bricks," pointing toward the surface in nice, orderly, maturing rows.

Sun damage causes chaos in the cells in this layer. It's as if the orderly brick wall were torn down by a storm and reassembled by a child who knows neither the correct height of a brick wall nor its correct arrangement. And that's exactly how radiaged epidermis looks under the microscope—like a dilapidated brick wall. The cells are of variable size and shape, prematurely detaching from each other. Disorder reigns.

But this battered brick wall is really capable of hurting you. The cells in it are not only disorderly, the nuclei are too large, irregular in size and shape, and very atypical—

Youth Alert!

The beautifully ordered arrangement of cells in the epidermis is effectively shattered by chronic radiaging. It's the equivalent of throwing old house paint onto a Rembrandt—a travesty!

---

in short, they're beginning to resemble cancer cells. These nuclei, as any freshman biology student knows, are the control centers that regulate cellular growth. This change is ominous, in that it indicates a tendency toward basal-cell and squamous-cell carcinomas, potentially perilous types of skin cancer.

Sunlight alters DNA in such a way that it no longer supports the ordinary orderly growth of the upper living layer of the skin, the epidermis. As the cells reproduce, mistakes are made in the copying process. The result is a landscape of premalignant changes.

These rough, hard spots of extreme disorganization in the skin (which lead to the second most common type of skin malignancy, called squamous-cell cancers) are called *actinic keratoses* (sun-induced scaly places), and as you'll see later, they are abolished by Retin-A. If you close your eyes and scan your forehead and nose with your fingers, you may be able to spot a few. If you feel anything scaly, that may be an actinic keratosis, and needs to be looked at by your dermatologist. Most of these keratoses are only cosmetically annoying, but those that become cancers can be locally destructive and can even kill by spreading to the other organs.

Pigment (skin coloration) is also greatly changed by radiaging. You've seen this before—a mottled, freckled look occurs with increased age. Chronic sun damage creates little piles of pigment under the epidermis, which we see on our arms and faces as ugly sun freckles. This results because the melanocytes, the cells that produce pigment,

═══════ *Youth Alert!* ═══════

Basal-cell and squamous-cell carcinomas are by far the most common cancers in this country. Over 600,000 cases of these nonmelanoma skin cancers develop in the United States every year.

become hyperactive and dump a lot of melanin unevenly into the basal layer. This leads to the stained, dirty, or murky look of radiaging skin.

It's not a pretty sight, as we all know. Each of us has seen this change hundreds of times—just think of the back of the hand of a sun-worshiping 70-year-old held next to the back of the hand of a teenager. Need I say more? And to add insult to injury, some dermatologists call these pigmented sunspots "senile freckles"! I long ago figured out it was much wiser to call them "barnacles on the ship of life," "birthday gifts," or even "*premature* age spots," in the hope that the patient will understand that the sun was the major problem that caused these ugly stains in the epidermis.

Sunlight, or some isolated fractions of it (the most damaging ones), does *not* just stop as soon as it strikes the dead layer of the skin. If it did, no one would ever have to worry about tanning—it just wouldn't work! That's because the color cells that make your skin pigment are deeper than that. It takes sunlight striking *them* to really produce a tan. Otherwise all Caucasians would be just as white as snow, instead of having the limitless variations in skin coloration that they have. Ultraviolet light zips right through the stratum corneum and epidermis into the deeper layers, where it damages the structural proteins (elastin and collagen) that make skin tough and durable. It's these structural proteins that you're testing when you do the pinch test.

Youth Alert!

Elastin is like a resilient network of supports for the skin. It allows the skin to snap back after stretching. Tough as it is, it is ruined by sunlight.

Elastin: The Rubber Bands of the Skin

Elastin is amazing stuff! It's a tough, nondissolvable protein that forms a network of resilient fibers. They stretch easily with every movement or deformation, but their really useful capability is that they enable the skin to snap back smartly. Without their elasticity, the skin would sag tremendously. That's what happens after they degenerate from excessive sun exposure.

With radiaging, your skin's beautiful architecture is blown to smithereens! And elastin is an early and terribly susceptible victim. From the first years of intense sunlight exposure, there is a loss of these delicate elastic fibers in the upper dermis. The fibers themselves first condense, and later disappear. This loosens the attachment to the dermis and allows the skin to stretch easily with any light force. Later, we'll talk about how sunscreens can prevent this destruction. For now, keep in mind that the *sun* causes all the damage, and that damage need not be incurred if we use a lot of what the American Cancer Society calls "sense in the sun."

Youth Alert!

Would you have ever thought that a pathologist looking at a skin specimen could actually tell your age by the amount of sun damage that you have in your skin? It's true!

Collagen and the Sun

Elastin makes up only about 5% of the dry weight of skin. Collagen makes up the great bulk and gives the skin its tensile strength. Arranged in bundles that constitute an interlocking network, collagen strongly resists stretching; it prevents the skin from tearing. Sturdy as it is, it can be totally destroyed by sunlight. If we could actually see the normal strands of collagen, they'd look like ropes—firm, sturdy, supporting ropes woven into a firm flooring of great mechanical strength. This all-important layer is what actually makes up the "leather" in a leather coat. And just as an old leather coat can dry up and crack with time and sunlight, so too can your orderly bundles of collagen degenerate into useless clumps. It's as if thousands of microscopic hand grenades had gone off in the midst of the beautiful lacework of collagen. The destruction is colossal. In the sun-damaged dermis, all that's left are mere fragments of what used to be a great network. When collagen is lost, the skin sags and hangs pitifully.

As it is assaulted by solar radiation, the collagen in many areas actually becomes reabsorbed, leaving less and less of this crucial supporting framework of the skin. In fact, enzymes are actually secreted to dissolve this support network. It's as if sunlight makes the dermis dissolve itself!

As the skin loses collagen, the dermis thins out year after year, causing loose skin where the taut, supple, resilient tissues of youth used to grow. The body tries to replace the collagen and elastin, but as long as sun exposure continues, it can only helplessly increase the surrounding ground substance, or gel, in which the fibers are suspended. This is a valiant effort, but increasing the ground substance is not the same as regrowing new collagen. It's like trying to build a wall out of mortar, with no bricks. In time, the skin no longer fits. There is too much of it and it is of very poor quality, loose and worn out.

Youth Alert!

Chronic sun exposure causes horrendous damage to the skin. The worst is the huge loss of collagen, depriving the skin of its tensile strength.

Until Retin-A came along, only strict sun avoidance and a large dose of time would even *begin* to heal some of the damage to the collagen layer. Research has shown that within a matter of several weeks of sun avoidance, irradiated skin can be made to heal *some* of the intense damage.

Retin-A, as we'll discuss later, greatly speeds up this natural repair process and extends it much deeper into the lower reaches of the skin, where almost all the severe damage is or has been done. The cells that ordinarily repair minor radiaging damage, the fibroblasts, can repair some damage on their own and become stimulated to produce more collagen under the influence of Retin-A.

Sun Squeezes Out the Skin's Lifeblood

Collagen and elastin are victims of sun damage, but so are other vital skin structures lying within its collagen framework. Among them are the blood vessels that provide nourishment to all strata of the skin. Some of the

---

Youth Alert!

With increasing sun exposure, the beautiful skin of your youth begins to look like a junkyard full of old dilapidated bricks. To rebuild it, you must first consider staying out of the sun for an extended time, which will permit your body's own defenses to repair and rebuild some of the damage.

===== *Youth Alert!* =====

Why do many sun-damaged people look paler than their age-matched counterparts? Radiaging destroys the skin blood vessels. The skin begins to look deathly white.

worst victims of chronic radiation damage, they are slashed to shreds as that damage takes place. In fact, in radiaged skin, the number of blood vessels dwindles dramatically. They become sparse, distorted, and irregular so that, looking at the skin in cross section, one wonders how it could even survive with such an infinitesimal blood supply.

The tiny remaining blood supply of radiaged skin does more than restrict its nourishment. The skin actually *looks* paler, as the very lifeblood is squeezed out of it! The glow of youth results from a rich blood supply. In sun-damaged skin, the blood supply is almost extinguished. In the office, dermatologists actually *see* this pallor in the facial skin of those with severe radiaging. The skin looks virtually lifeless. But Retin-A, researchers have found, can restore and regrow some of those vital blood vessels.

Adhesive Tape: A Simple Lesson in Sun Damage

As if the loss of blood vessels were not enough, the radiaged epidermis slowly flattens and loses the interlocking projections that help anchor it to the dermis. You can think of this like the balding of a set of tires: Without the necessary tread to maintain traction between the tires and the road surface, slipping and sliding occur, sometimes resulting in disaster. What's the day-to-day meaning of this effacement of the attachment "treads" between skin strata? Skin fragility.

As a medical student, I started IVs on every age group of patients. When I removed tape from the arms of people who were not only young but undamaged by the sun, the tape pulled at the hairs a little, but the skin was never injured by it. But I noticed over the years of working on the medical wards that people with a lot of sun damage— farmers, passionate gardeners, avid sailors, professional tanners—would react a lot differently to the tape. Besides not even *having* as much hair on their skin (probably an intrinsic, or time-related, change, not due to sun damage), the skin itself would often separate and tear right away with the tape! It took but a couple of episodes like this to teach me to examine for radiaging. And I learned an experienced physician's tip quickly, of writing an order in huge red letters on the chart of any such patient to "USE *NO* TAPE ON THIS PATIENT'S SKIN!" All bandages could easily be secured by wrapping gently with gauze, instead of tape.

Bruising

But it was not until years later, at the start of my dermatology residency, that I learned of another prominent sign of the sun's devastation: bleeding into the skin of sun-exposed areas with very minor trauma. We used to call that "senile purpura" (age bruising), and most assuredly some do get this just by aging (and from occasional other causes, like alcoholism, liver diseases, and steroids), but for the most part, we would have been much more accurate to call it "solar purpura," or "sun bruising," because that's the real cause.

If you consider the blood vessels in the skin as railroad tracks, and their collagen support network as the railroad ties, you'll better understand what happens when sun degrades collagen. It's equivalent to splitting each of the railroad ties into a thousand toothpicks, wiping out some altogether, and then expecting them to support the weight of a fully loaded train! No way! If the train passed over the track, the rails would twist and break, just as the blood vessels in the skin would rupture with even the lightest mechanical force.

With chronic exposure and many of these bruises, the arm skin often takes on a muddy brown tone, as if stained with time itself. Some of these marks left after "sun bruising" actually are stains, of a sort, almost like tattoos, since the blood pigment that causes them is like an iron stain of rust deep down in the skin. The iron comes from hemoglobin, the lifesaving oxygen carrier in the blood. In the center of each hemoglobin molecule is one molecule of iron. When the blood leaks out of a blood vessel, the red blood cells eventually break up and leave their hemoglobin pigment just below the skin. The hemoglobin degrades through several steps (that's what causes the various shades of color in a bruise, as it resolves over several weeks—blue-black to blue to green to green-yellow to pale yellow), ending up with the deposition of the iron in the dermis.

You know what iron pigments look like if you've ever seen a rust stain: brownish red. And unfortunately, this stain is sometimes thought to be permanent. Since there is no good system for eliminating this color from the skin, you must just wait for the color to fade. Often, in adults, it does fade slightly, but the tattooed color can remain, and it's extremely difficult to remove with current techniques except when Retin-A is appropriately used. By increasing the blood supply, Retin-A promotes removal of the iron pigment.

In my first book, *Skin Secrets*, I talked about a partial solution to this bruising problem: three- to five-minute pressure on minor trauma sites, and taking a vitamin containing zinc and vitamin C. But it would be much better if we used an ounce of prevention and avoided sun damage and trauma to the skin instead of a pound of cure (or an eventual pound of Retin-A!) on that same skin.

Youth Alert!

In one study, only 90 exposures to ultraviolet light were necessary to cause severe sun damage. Some children could get that in a single summer!

All these changes, says Dr. Albert Kligman, father of Retin-A, occur only in radiaged skin, *never* in normal non-sun-exposed aging of skin. Sure makes one consider sun-screens more seriously, doesn't it? But how much sun damage is necessary to produce changes like this? There's an interesting study to demonstrate exactly how *little* damage is required.

10 Weeks to Cancer

In a study of hairless mice, reported in the *Journal of the American Academy of Dermatology*, Drs. Lorraine and Albert Kligman treated the mice with ultraviolet light for only 10 weeks before tumors appeared in the skin of every mouse. Just think of that! Only 10 weeks to cancer. And in another experiment, mice given just three treatments per week for 30 weeks were all found to have serious radiaging changes, consisting of most of the defects I've already mentioned, including collagen and elastin damage after treatment far *less* in severity than the average vacationer gets in a few years! And think of our teenagers. A kid could conceivably get that much sunlight in a single summer! No wonder I've taken basal-cell skin cancers off the skin of even 18-year-old sunbathing addicts! If only we could get the general population to realize how *little* sun damage is really necessary to cause a problem, especially in light-skinned persons.

Realize, too, that this same type of damage has been found to occur in mice treated with UVA radiation, too, which is the same type our young people are flocking to in what I call the "tanning coffins" (tanning beds). The damage the kids get in these devices is up to 1,000 times greater than natural sunlight because the radiation is so intense. Tanning parlors accelerate radiaging and can damage the eyes as well. They are a menace to skin health.

The Skin Tries to Repair Itself

The Kligmans discovered that radiaged collagen will slowly be repaired, if left undamaged for a long enough time. This "repair zone " started to show up at 15 weeks in the damaged mice, but the Kligmans found that treating these mice with Retin-A resulted in rapid formation of new collagen in only 10 weeks, fully one-third faster than nature left to its own course. Findings such as these led to the idea that radiaging changes such as the Kligmans had seen reversed and repaired in mice might also be reversed in human skin. Dr. Albert Kligman's landmark photographs showed many remarkable improvements in sun-damaged skin treated with Retin-A.

How Retin-A Repairs Your Skin

At the start of this chapter, I told you how important it was to understand the biological basis for what we see on our skin as wrinkles. Now that you've seen how severe that damage can be, let's take a look layer by layer to see what changes are wrought by Retin-A.

First, it's easy to notice that something very powerful has acted on the dead layer of the skin. Normally arranged in a loose basket-weave network of dead cells, it appears tremendously compacted down into a narrow but solid structure. We don't know why this occurs, but it is very important, and may account for some of the sun sensitivity that you'll read about in Chapter 4.

================= *Youth Alert!* =================

Retin-A has been shown to return true order to the skin's growth pattern. Thus it eliminates many superficial effects of radiaging—even potential skin cancers!

And the "brick wall" is also rebuilt, this time by a master mason! The dilapidated cells of the irradiated epidermis, which had been irregular in size and shape, showing shrunken, abnormal nuclei, now become uniform and well-ordered again, looking like the epidermis of a teenager (an un-sun-damaged teenager, that is!). And the epidermis, previously just a couple of cells high after this much radiaging, now has quadrupled or quintupled in thickness! This means that millions of lazy, resting cells have been stimulated by Retin-A to divide, thickening up this topmost living layer of skin.

The disorganized cells that were slowly and inevitably changing into serious skin cancers are gone! Or rather, they are made to change back into the type of well-regulated, well-ordered cells we'd like to see when we look closely at the epidermis. This reversion of skin that was premalignant back to normal is called *differentiation*. We'll be talking about differentiation from time to time throughout this book, but basically, Retin-A causes cells to behave the way they *ought* to act.

A cell, in some respects, is like a developing, growing person, who starts off life as an immature child, then changes, or "differentiates," into an adult who acts responsibly and normally, in a socially controlled fashion. Later, if that adult ages and contracts a degenerative disease like Alzheimer's, he may regress to a more childlike behavior pattern. For the skin, Retin-A could be said to be like a cure for the disease of sun-induced old age. It can be described as a "normalizing" influence on the skin.

This change is the main reason dermatologists prescribe it. Even though it's nice to get the cosmetic result of wrinkle reversal, it's even nicer to reverse these premalignant alterations in the epidermis. In other words, it's what I call a "win, win, win" situation—the patient wins twice, by getting to see and talk with the dermatologist and get his skin checked, and by reversing some of the minor lines on the face. The doctor wins by knowing that he has reversed many of the premalignant changes in the skin that may have sooner or later become a problem of major proportions, just as it had in thousands of patients with radiaging in the days prior to Retin-A. And in many patients he can actually elicit the promise to avoid further intentional damage.

Does it really get patients out of the sun? I can only tell you this—in 15 years of dermatologic practice, I've preached for thousands of hours about the dangers of sun exposure with only moderate results, until the recent discoveries about Retin-A. Now, for the first time, I've got a real tool, which is so coveted by patients that they will amend their damaging tanning habits!

Dr. Kligman says, and I verify this daily with my patients in the office who are using it, that the changes after a patient *starts* Retin-A are the most dramatic, and that we often would not have suspected all that much damage existed at the onset of therapy and during the initial examination. In other words, people can be significantly radiaged and not even know it! A skin beautiful to the naked eye may be horrible under the microscope.

I can personally vouch for that, because after starting the drug myself, a premalignant keratosis appeared on my nose that I never even *suspected* I had, prior to starting the drug. At eight months into my treatment, two more lesions appeared! This meant that even I had some premalignant sunspots, as fanatic as I am about sun exposure! But it was good that they appeared—I finally realized on a personal level what the sun can do to a person. The nice thing about Retin-A is that it wipes out these

---

Youth Alert!

Some ultraviolet damage is present in almost every white young adult, even though it's not apparent clinically. But you'll see it pop out after a few weeks or months on Retin-A. We should not be fooled or complacent about good-looking skin.

---

bad spots with slow, chronic use. The spots on my nose reddened a little and the Retin-A just melted them away in a matter of several weeks. In other words, Retin-A flushed them out and destroyed them before my very eyes.

But the dead layer and the epidermis are not the only places Kligman, at his Philadelphia Clinic for Aging Skin, noted a change in Retin-A patients. Both the dermal-epidermal junction and the dermis itself were partially but significantly repaired by this drug. The junction regained some of its "tread"—the grooves that kept the topmost epidermis from sliding right off the dermis below.

Fading Brown Spots: A Retin-A Specialty

One of the biggest complaints of patients with sun-aged skin is the appearance of "pigmentation brown spots," as they say on the TV commercials. If you develop these, you

---

Youth Alert!

Beneficial changes in human skin can be seen on a microscopic level in as little as 10 days on Retin-A. New, fresh, younger collagen just pours into the treated areas.

---

can apply all the over-the-counter pigment lighteners you want, for *years* even, and you won't budge them. But in a few short months, Retin-A can erase them so well that you may see "lines of cutoff" where you stopped applying the medicine, as Dr. John Vorhees observed in his extensive studies of the anti-radiaging effect of the drug.

One of my own patients, a man in his 40s with a lot of sun damage on his Celtic skin, started using Retin-A for the damage on his chest, which was just covered with premalignant sunspots and sun freckles. As you already know, Retin-A will remove sunspots with time, but I didn't think much about the sun freckles when he came in the first time for Retin-A. He used it on his entire chest for a few months, following the program you'll learn about in Chapter 4. When he returned to my office, there was an amazingly clear-cut line on the shoulder between the stained, sun-damaged skin of his arm and the fresh new chest skin. It was as if someone had scrubbed off the radiaging.

A Different Kind of Sun Bumps: Whiteheads and Blackheads

We all know about the wrinkling and laxity of the skin the sun produces. But have you thought about some of its other side effects? One of the problems we see most often is the creation of "sun blackheads," or comedones on the faces of the chronically sun-exposed. These troublesome spots are usually seen in those with the worst sun damage and severe wrinkling, called "end-stage" damage, because at this late date it cannot all be reversed by *any* method.

You may have seen these spots on people with sun damage. They look like large blackheads and whiteheads, located chiefly around the eyes and temples. They are found frequently in those who work outdoors or in oily environments such as machine shops and restaurants.

Youth Alert!

Age- and sun-related blackheads and whiteheads can be effectively treated with Retin-A when used carefully.

The good news is that these sun blackheads can be helped dramatically by Retin-A. We'll be talking more in Chapter 4 on exactly how to increase the dosage to tolerance to remove these very tough spots.

The Downside of Retin-A

What's the downside to Retin-A as an anti-aging drug? While the upside greatly outweighs the disadvantages, Kligman did notice certain problems. First, for anyone over the age of 25, when the oil output of the skin begins to slow, the skin does tend to be drier. By thinning the dead layer, Retin-A adds to this drying effect, which may show as fine peeling and may be rough to the touch. This leads to a loss of water from the epidermis, an area normally well shielded from evaporation by the retained dead layer above. The water loss is at least doubled in areas treated with Retin-A. What does this mean for you in your quest for a "Youth Miracle"? *Dry skin*. And that's why I'll devote a good many words to teaching you how to solve this problem while on Retin-A. However, the skin does tend to improve as the skin adjusts to Retin-A.

Also, because Retin-A causes some irritation at the start, any skin is more likely to become sunburned after short exposure. Therefore, caution is necessary. The initial sensitivity to the sun does lessen with time and continued use of the drug, however. See Chapter 4 for further information on side effects.

Retin-A Won't Work for Everything

Dr. Kligman's pioneer testing of Retin-A in radiaged skin did show some things that the drug would *not* clear up: Moles, which grow much bumpier with age, showed no change, nor did fibrous bumps in the skin called fibromas or the brownish, waxy "warts" of aging called seborrheic keratoses. Kligman and most of us in dermatology have noted that patients often request removal of these "barnacles on the ship of life," as I call them, after their skin has greatly improved in quality from Retin-A use. They seem to feel that if they already look better and have tolerated the side effects of Retin-A, why not go all the way and get the signs of TMB (too many birthdays) removed too!

Interestingly, I have one (and only one) patient in my hundreds who have used Retin-A who claims that *more* tiny skin tags appear on the neck when she's on the medicine. These are the tiny fleshy excrescences that form on the necks and underarms in many people who have the genetic trait for them. And in fact, on seeing her from time to time, she does indeed seem to have more of them, but this could be coincidental with her normal aging process (she's about 40). She claims, however, that they fade and go away when she's *not* using the Retin-A. It's something clinical dermatologists will have to watch for as we start to treat more and more women and men in this age group. It would hardly be the first time that we've noticed new findings when a drug is used for a novel indication.

When to Start Retin-A

Here are a few recommendations from Dr. Kligman's studies on Retin-A and from my day-to-day office practice. The medicine is best used as a *preventive*. Why wait till the horse is stolen to close the barn door? It's much better

---

Youth Alert!

The best way to think of Retin-A? As a preventive, not as a mechanism to reverse already intense damage. In other words, the earlier you start, the better!

---

to *prevent* the damage than it is to try to reverse it. And, as I've indicated, that includes a modification of your sun exposure habits. However, there is this caveat: Starting Retin-A to prevent radiaging must be approached cautiously, because undamaged skin is much more sensitive to Retin-A irritation.

Starting Retin-A early may be very important, because the microscopic changes in the skin start as early as 10 to 15 years before they can be seen. Naturally, the changes are more dramatic in the older, more radiaged population.

Because it's a long-term treatment and perhaps a lifetime commitment, Kligman advises light-skinned people (Scotch, Irish, Nordic, Celtic, fair-skinned, blue-eyed, red-haired, and natural blonds) to start Retin-A in their 20s, and all others (and that's most of us) in their 30s or 40s.

Not having heard this advice, I missed the suggested age of starting the drug by just a couple of years. Now I, too, am trying to catch up with the clock, rather than having kept up with it from my early 30s. If you've passed these "ideal" ages for starting Retin-A, you can still start it and expect a good effect. There's no hard-and-fast rule

---

Youth Alert!

Retin-A cannot do its job overnight. The Retin-A program demands a lot of fortitude. Because improvement is gradual, some people are skeptical. However, it will work in almost everybody, given a little diligence and time.

---

about starting it at these ages—these are just *optimum* times to try to prevent and reverse radiaging. In fact, the majority of my patients start the medicine in their 40s, 50s, and 60s.

When I described the effects of Retin-A treatment to a dive partner on a Caribbean trip, he said, "I'm not sure that whole process doesn't sound a little like putting a 40-year paint job on a 4-year car! After all, we're only designed to be on this planet for about a hundred years!" He had definitely missed the point. Most of us want to *stay* as young-looking as possible as long into those intended hundred years as possible!

Finally, no chapter on the research findings about Retin-A could be complete without mentioning that Retin-A is just one of virtually *hundreds* of retinoids, or vitamin A–related compounds, that are currently under study for use in skin therapy. It indeed could be true that the future will hold pleasant surprises for dermatologists and patients alike. Should you wait for these new drugs and delay Retin-A? Don't consider that until you read all the marvelous things Retin-A can do for you right here and now.

3

Wrinkles: How They Can Happen, and What You Can Do About Them

When a 40-year-old woman leans into her mirror and finds the first wrinkle, that's a disaster.

—Albert M. Kligman, MD

We'll be talking a lot about wrinkles in this book, and it's important that the term *wrinkle* be understood. The Random House Dictionary of the English Language defines a wrinkle as "a small furrow or crease in the skin, especially of the face, as from aging or frowning."

At first you might say that a wrinkle is a wrinkle is a wrinkle—what's the difference? In fact, there are many different types of wrinkles, and many different causes for them. The purpose of this chapter is to explain them better, and to tell you something about how scientists are redefining them, in the hopes of treating them more successfully.

Six Causes of Wrinkles and How to Fight Them

The best classification of wrinkles and their causes comes from Dr. Samuel Stegman, associate professor of der-

---

══ *Youth Alert!* ══

*Wrinkles originate in different ways and are not all
the same. Their common background, however, is
sun damage.*

---

matology and dermatologic surgery at the University of
California–San Francisco. In an interview published in
the October 1988 *Dialogues in Dermatology*, Dr. Stegman
reviewed what he called the six major factors causing
wrinkles on the human face. Using them, a clinician can
determine in a few minutes whether a face lift is needed
to *redrape* the skin, or an acid peel to *resurface* the skin, or
a filler substance, such as collagen or silicone, to *recontour*
the skin. You can take this book to a mirror after you've
read this chapter and analyze your own wrinkles—at least
preliminarily—before visiting the dermatologist or cosmetic surgeon.

1. *Chronologic aging* is the factor that causes the droopy
texture and looseness of the skin with the passage of time.
Even Dr. Kligman's famous monk who was 90 and looked
50, by avoiding sunlight and leading a contemplative and
calm lifestyle, had some drooping. That's inevitable.

For these saggy areas, plastic surgery may be the only
way to redrape the skin and flatten some of the folds that
are associated with aging. Heredity, too, plays a role here.

2. *Loss of underlying support tissues* with age. This is
not commonly recognized by nonprofessionals, but it does
definitely occur with time and aging, probably more significantly in women than in men. This accounts for the
"purse string" wrinkles around the mouth, for instance;
the mouth skin actually becomes too large for the mouth
opening as the underlying fat and muscle recede with age.
Of course, other factors come into play, such as smoking
and the presence of dentures, which can cause erosion of
the bony ridges that usually hold the teeth. Also, as people

age, you've probably noticed some sinking in of the cheeks and temples with time, another effect of loss of the tissues below the skin.

Here, prevention may be the key. Such measures as keeping your teeth in good shape so that you never have to lose them will help. Almost everyone who has dentures has a greater problem with this loss of substance in the upper lip, where the purse string wrinkles first appear. In future years, when the safety and efficacy of fat replacement (fat reimplantation) are established, this may become the method of choice for restoring the substance of the underlying tissues, but as yet, this has not proved to be safe.

3. *Sun damage*. This is the most destructive, but also the most preventable, of all the forces that cause wrinkles. As the sun progressively destroys the upper dermis, that layer tends to become thinner, less resilient, and more foldable. Think of it like this: If you were trying to fold paper, wouldn't it be a lot easier to fold a thin layer, say, 2 or 3 sheets, rather than 50 or 60? The thin, easy folds correspond to skin radiaged by the sun, while the thicker skin corresponds to skin that has been protected or partially restored to youthful thickness by Retin-A. As we would expect, more wrinkles form when this folding occurs repeatedly, as it does on the face.

Preventing sun damage and radiaging, even among sun worshipers, is as easy as grabbing a hat and applying the highest-protection sunscreen.

4. *Movement-related changes*. Interesting, isn't it, that no other species communicates with its face so intently, so elegantly. A single raised eyebrow, or a wink of an eye, or a frown, or a sidelong glance occasionally tells entire stories all by itself. Yet our penalty for that subtle communicative skill is that the skin overlying the muscles that make those expressions is folded virtually millions of times in our lifetime. I consider it remarkable that our skin is *so* durable that it can survive this with only a few wrinkles.

We all recognize these creases. They start around the eyes (crow's feet) in the 40s, and with time get progressively more pronounced. They are also the ones that form the little parentheses that enclose the mouth. Some dermatologists call them "man's penalty for learning how to smile," because species that don't smile (and that's all the others) just don't have them!

Dr. Stegman notes that we all smile and express ourselves at all ages of life, but it's not until the tissues themselves are assaulted by external factors like sun damage that these creases begin to become permanent. If you think of how often babies and children smile, laugh, and otherwise express themselves, this theory explains it exactly.

But also ask yourself: Is it really necessary, to use the words of dermatologist Dr. Wilma Bergfeld, to express all our thoughts by forming our faces into a "Chicago Bears Grimace"? Not at all.

I thought about this years ago while starting my career in dermatology, studying some of the TV personalities we see every day in our living rooms. Just watch them closely, and you'll see ample examples of all types of forehead creases. You can see why, if you watch some of the interviewers on the news or on talk shows. When the host is under pressure with an important guest, he wrinkles that area of his forehead intensely with each question. It's an indicator of stress and concentration, pure and simple.

Interestingly, it's also this crease that a skilled poker player learns to eliminate from his facial repertoire as soon as he can, so that he can bluff his opponent successfully. He knows, as do the rest of us, that these expressions tell volumes to those who watch us. So we all need to become better "poker faces" if we want to eliminate and prevent this type of wrinkle!

How do we go about about it? The answer sounds a lot easier than it is: Stop using your face for every expression of your internal feelings. "Sure," I can hear you saying, "that's easy for *you* to say! But how do I change a lifetime habit?" I can only tell you that it *is* possible. Ever since I

Youth Alert!

If you must show emotional concern over every-thing, try to do it verbally instead of scrunching up your face to show expression—adopt a poker face and you'll show less wrinkling!

gave this some thought years ago while still a dermatology resident, I have concentrated on *not* needlessly wrinkling up my face. Of course, I'll admit to being very strict about avoiding the sun and using Retin-A, too, as you already know, but I'm convinced that those who give the smooth-faced approach a try can really see results. In fact, some investigators, like Dr. Stegman, believe that the wrinkles actually *do* recede with time, as the face is steadily relaxed. Stegman relates the commonly observed fact that a person who has a stroke and has lax musculature on one side of the face quickly loses his wrinkles on that side too—a result of loss of muscle movements.

Another striking example is Dr. Kligman's photo of the 90-year-old monk who had nary a wrinkle, due to his stoical lifestyle. There's no doubt that such a relaxed face can virtually eliminate expression-caused wrinkles. Yoga and other such disciplines can also result in a passive, less wrinkled face.

5. *Gravity*. This inexorable force draws our bodies *down* with time. Or at least it draws *parts* down, or makes loose and floppy the skin of the eyelids, jowls, chin, breasts, and so forth.

It is probably also responsible for the apparent elongation of the earlobes and nose with time, along with the second factor, shrinking away of the underlying tissues. The effect is to make the skin *look* like it's getting bigger than is needed to cover the face.

Unless we want to spend half our time on our heads, or set some longevity record in outer space, we'll not really be able to combat this in any way except surgery. This is where the classic redraping procedures are necessary to refit the skin to the face.

6. *Sleep creases*. I had often wondered whether sleeping eight hours on a pillow could cause changes in the facial skin, ever since I first slept on a hard old kapok pillow someone gave me on a camping trip long ago. It was either that or my arm, and I mistakenly chose the hard pillow. I awoke the next morning with half of my face numb! It had "gone to sleep" due to the intense pressure of the firm pillow. There is no doubt whatsoever that sleep pressures on sun-damaged facial skin can cause deep folds in the skin.

You can spot these wrinkles easily. Try this test to see whether you or your spouse has these creases: Have a person lie down with a firm pillow, as he would while he is sleeping. If you get close, you may see vertical lines on the face in the areas of the temples, running in some cases from the temples almost all the way down the face to the lower cheeks. Note that expression lines are never oriented in this direction. They always run the way the lines form if you look into the mirror and give yourself a "Chicago Bears Grimace." You just can't make a vertical line on the sides of your face with any expression you can dream of. In children, sleep creases disappear at breakfast. In adults, they are permanent.

But you don't really have to get these particular wrinkles at all. I'll give you Dr. Stegman's advice: Amend the way you sleep on your face! Try sleeping with the weight of your head centered over the ear area, instead of burying your face deeply into the pillow, or sleep on your back if you can. Make this the last thing you think of at night and the first thing you think of in the morning. Then, says Dr. Stegman, you'll begin to slowly change the weight distribution for your head over the next several months. This done, most of your sleep creases will melt away. Chinese ladies knew this thousands of years ago; they slept on concave porcelain pillows—on their backs.

Now here's *my* addition to this tip. I heartily agree with Dr. Stegman, but I would advise one important investment on your part: *the best and softest goosedown pillow you can get your hands on.* Don't spare any expense here, and you'll be rewarded a thousand times by the appearance of your face. Remember my story about the borrowed kapok pillow on my camping trip? Just think of the effect 20,000 nights of sleeping with your face crammed into a hard pillow can have. Maybe someone will invent an air jet pillow someday that will let us rest without touching anything, but until that happens, the supersoft down pillow is your best choice.

If you'll pay attention to the six factors that cause wrinkles on your face, you have every chance of having skin as unwrinkled as Dr. Kligman's monk, all your life.

What Won't Help Wrinkles

We also know some things that won't help wrinkles: massages and facials, mudpacks, masks, gels, glazes, all sorts of food that are applied to the skin, and even moisturizers, which do nothing whatsoever to correct the wrinkles except to make them *appear* better by softening the dead layer of the skin for a few minutes. This is the reason many cosmetic companies have been able to successfully modify their advertising to state that "Cream X will make you *appear* instantly younger!" Ridiculous! All it does is slightly moisturize the skin for a few minutes to hours, plumping it up so that the furrows are a little less visible. This is mainly an optical effect and not a real treatment. There is *nothing* on the over-the-counter market today that will help wrinkles in any permanent, or even long-lasting, way. You could do the same thing or better using Crisco as a facial moisturizer than by spending hundreds of dollars on the plethora of hoaxes these companies are trying to sell you.

The same principle applies to night creams, which women have been indoctrinated to use every night of their lives. There is no conceivable reason to use a cream on the face nightly (except Retin-A, of course), unless you're dry-skinned and want to moisturize a little before bed. But don't expect it to change your skin lines, wrinkles, and folds one iota—it won't!

Cell Turnover and Skin Irritation

Cosmetic chemists have gone hog-wild over the new Retin-A findings and have struggled to obtain the same results with "anti-aging" cosmetics. To do this, they have centered on a concept called the "cell turnover rate." They claim that the real problem in wrinkled, aging skin is that the cells in the epidermis were not replicating fast enough. They used a staining test, called the dansyl chloride test (first devised by Kligman), to demonstrate that the skin cells could indeed be made to divide faster. Dansyl chloride is a fluorescent dye (visible only under black light) that stains only the dead layer of the skin. As the cells are shed at the surface, the dye gradually disappears in a measurable length of time; when the glow disappears completely, the dead layer has fully reproduced itself from top to bottom.

The fact is that mild irritants will also stimulate cell turnover by increasing nonspecifically the multiplication of epidermal cells. *Any* irritated skin will make cells more rapidly to try to repair the damage, regardless of the stimulus. The question is, is slow cell turnover what causes the signs of aging? And is a rapid cell turnover the key to staying young?

The answer is uncertain, but there are some reasons that may make you want to avoid such preparations. Certainly almost every function of the skin decreases with

Youth Alert!

Beware of cosmetic systems that claim to renew your skin by increasing "cell turnover." You may just be wearing out your skin or causing slow but persistent damage.

age, but wrinkles are made by different forces altogether, summarized in the six Stegman Factors. Skin cells in culture, such as those in the epidermis, do not live immortally even under the best of laboratory circumstances. They appear to have a finite number of cell divisions before they just wear out! So these cosmetics that claim to stimulate the turnover of the epidermis worry some of us dermatologists because they may just cause *earlier* aging in the skin, not later aging. After a long time the effects could be negative—worse wrinkling! The bottom line on such products: Avoid them. Some of them cause low-grade irritation that can damage skin after decades of use.

Retin-A works by a totally different mechanism to actually unlock cells that are in the resting phase: It releases them into the "proliferative compartment" of actively dividing cells, and that's exactly what we'd like to obtain to rejuvenate the skin. But we know Retin-A has many other desirable effects in addition to correcting cell turnover.

Everything Goes Down with Age

We should talk about some of the functions of the skin that decrease with age and help create the types of wrinkles that Dr. Stegman has so beautifully classified. These include the skin's response to injury—we all know that healing slows down in the elderly. The classic example of this is the common leg ulcer, which, even when small, can take months to heal, with thousands of dollars spent in

care. Yet the same ulcer in a young, healthy per-
uld rapidly be resurfaced. In the laboratory, blisters heal much faster in young skin than in old skin.

Barrier function decreases with age, too. That means
the skin is much more susceptible to injury than the same
location of intact skin in a younger person.

Chemicals and drugs put on the skin are slower to be
carried away than in younger skin. This may be related to
the slower circulation in the skin of the elderly, due to the
loss of many small blood vessels. Older people seem to
tolerate Retin-A better than younger ones because their
skin is less easily inflamed. However, dry scaling skin is
more frequent in the elderly.

The skin's immunity decreases with age, too. It's harder
to sensitize an older person to any of the common substances to which the young become so easily allergic. For
example, fewer older adults are allergic to poison ivy,
including those who were previously allergic to it. That
means that they've lost some of their immune competence
with time. Many studies bear out this age decline in
immune functions. These changes are relative and no cause
for alarm.

Sensations cannot be felt as well in aging skin. We see
this quite often in the office when we freeze premalignant
spots on the skin. Equivalent freezes would hurt the
younger patient much more. Many is the time that I never
see a flinch in an alert older patient. Maybe that stoicism
comes with age, but it happens too often to believe that.
That skin is less sensitive owing to loss of finer nerve
endings.

We know that chronic sun damage destroys the blood
vessels in the upper dermis, drastically decreasing the
blood flow in the skin. This accounts for the loss of the
normal pinkish, healthy color of the skin. It also has a
bearing on thermoregulation, the ability to control heat
in the body through the body's air conditioning unit, the
skin.

It would be hard to dream up a more efficient way to control body temperature at a fixed level. In the summer, we open up our skin blood vessels wide and exude heat through our reddened skin. Vast amounts of extra heat produced by exercise and weather can be eliminated this way. And sweating is the evaporative cooling unit of the skin, one of the most efficient self-protective mechanisms of the body. Have you ever seen the evaporative coolers people have in the Southwest? These coolers operate on the basis of the area's low humidity. These units are like huge mats that are bathed with water, which constantly evaporates and loses heat when it does so. Air is passed through the cool areas to discharge heat and bring coolness into the home. It works fabulously if all is well with the unit, provided the humidity is low. However, during the rainy season the humidity goes up and the ability of the unit to cool the home decreases miserably.

We could equate the aging human with an evaporative cooling unit that has lost some of its ability to cool. That's why it's so vital to make sure the elderly have a cool environment in the summer. Hot weather is a great stress for old people. They cannot eliminate heat as well as the rest of us because of the lack of efficient circulation in their skins and the drastic decrease in sweating. They should be encouraged to seek cool basements if they lack air conditioners.

No one claims that Retin-A reverses all these functional declines. But we know it can help blood flow by inducing growth of new vessels in the upper layers of the skin, producing a rosy color in the facial skin.

Most of these age-related changes, such as decreased sensitivity of the skin, loss of allergic potential, and decreased sweating will not be noticeably helped by using Retin-A, but Retin-A does increase the number of new blood vessels in radiaged skin, and perhaps encourages better heat regulation in the areas where it is used.

4

The Day-to-Day Use of Retin-A

The day you teach 'em how to use a toothbrush, get the sunscreens on 'em, because it's the young in whom the damage is the greatest.
—*Albert M. Kligman, MD*

A few months ago, a patient of mine came red-faced and tearful into my consultation room. When she looked up at me, I could see she had swollen, red eyes, which reminded me of someone who had recently gone through some terrible tragedy and had cried her eyes out. But I knew Jenny very well, having been a family friend, and I knew of no family disaster.

"Jenny, what's happening?" I asked, as she kept her head down, continually wiping her eyes.

"I just didn't want you to see *this*!" she exclaimed, as her head rose and she looked into my eyes. I was aghast! Her face looked as red as fire, and her eyes were swollen almost shut.

"Hmmm . . ." I said, trying not to sound too alarmed. (That's the sound doctors make when they're *really* alarmed about something.) "Looks like you grabbed the steel wool instead of your washcloth this morning. What caused this?"

"Retin-A!" exclaimed Jenny. "I'll never use that stuff again!" Her words reminded me of the words of a well-respected dermatologist I had encountered during my training. I asked him why he didn't use more Retin-A in acne therapy. "Best stuff I ever saw for keeping my phone ringing, Joe," he said. "The kids keep calling me to ask why their faces look like raw beefsteaks while they're using it!" That very statement caused me to become overcautious about the medicine for many years of dermatologic practice. Learning about the side effects of Retin-A and using the drug extensively in my practice changed all that.

But I had to find out more about Jenny's rash. Where had she gotten the Retin-A? Looking back over my records, I saw that *I* had never prescribed it for her. Also, I had to know what else she was using. Had some other topical agent reacted with it, causing the irritation? We often see this interaction with skin products. When I pursued this possibility, she told me she had gotten a prescription for the *high-strength gel* from a cardiologist next door whom she had also known for years. Besides this, she was using nothing different, and as far as facial treatments and lotions went, the Retin-A was all she was applying.

"How often do you use it—nightly, or every other night?"

"Oh, more often than that," she replied. "You know how impatient I am. I wanted my wrinkles to go away right away, so I've been applying it *three to five times a day!*"

"Incredible!" I gasped. "Did you know that this stuff's an acid?"

She didn't, of course, nor did she know very much at all about the medicine. She learned the hard way. And in fact, that's the way most women (and men) learn about this potentially fantastic medicine: through trial and error—mostly error.

Obviously, one needs the correct instructions for *any* medicine, including Retin-A. Retin-A is a prescription *medicine*, and a strong one at that. You wouldn't go to your neurologist and ask for a seizure medicine without getting proper instructions for taking it, would you? Of course not. But you'd be astounded at how many patients who

Youth Alert!

If you want correct instructions in using a medicine, first get the medicine from the appropriate doctor—in the case of Retin-A, a dermatologist—then make sure you get the correct concentration of the medicine and follow his instructions conscientiously. You are the principal player in the Retin-A theater!

have come to me with complications or complaints about Retin-A without ever having gotten anything like proper instructions for its use.

I'm reminded here of the news bulletins describing the studies that proved the efficacy of Retin-A. Those studies, released in January 1988, were followed, as you already know, by the loudest commotion ever engendered by news of a new medicine. On one of the major networks, correspondents interviewed several dermatologists about the use of this drug for reversal of radiaging. During the demonstration of how to apply it, a patient was shown slathering on about a *tablespoonful* of Retin-A cream to the *upper eyelid*! That was bad enough. What was worse yet was that the subject was an elderly gentleman with "farmer's skin," with devastating wrinkles and sagging. His skin was *so* severely sun-damaged that a gallon of Retin-A a *day* wouldn't help a great deal. In other words, this, the *first* introduction that many viewers had to this medicine, was wrong in at least three ways: wrong *subject*, wrong *area of application*, and wrong *quantity*.

Jenny had watched just that "informational" spot, and applied the drug to her eyelids on its advice—thus her trouble. Needless to say, I put her on the right track by stopping the cream for a few days and starting it again when all the inflammation had subsided. Today she's back on the medicine and using it effectively.

In the ensuing weeks, I found many men and women who got their first inklings of how to use Retin-A from

====== *Youth Alert!* ======

As Dr. J. Graham Smith Jr. told me, "Joe, if your patient does something wrong, it's often your fault for not explaining it correctly."

just such news items, and from physicians who knew nearly nothing about the drug except the name. These doctors had apparently forgotten the physician's prime directive: "Primum non nocere"—first, do no *harm*!

Treating Jenny's troubles with Retin-A made me decide that Dr. Kligman, the father of Retin-A, is right when he says that about 30 *minutes* of explanation are required just to get a person off on the right foot when *starting* Retin-A, let alone the follow-up visits to the dermatologist to check on the progress of the treatment. The program I outline for you here is one of regular dermatologic care, not a one-time "get-the-cream-and-run" experience.

Starting Retin-A

All forms of Retin-A are not equal. There are several dosage formulations, and there's a *right* way for almost everybody to start on the right one for his complexion type. See Table 1 for a summary of those dosage forms and the patients for whom they are appropriate. Keep in mind

====== *Youth Alert!* ======

The real and too frequent tragedy in not getting the right instructions for using Retin-A is not that you may experience some of the side effects without understanding them—it's that you may stop using this medicine and be deprived of its benefits!

that these suggestions are derived from my extensive clinical experience with hundreds of patients who have used this drug under my close supervision. However, my experience may not match your individual one, and is in no way intended to serve as a hard and fast set of rules in the use of Retin-A for radiaging! I watch each and every patient very closely on this potent medicine, and I wouldn't suggest any less attentive care for you. Use this table *as a guideline only*. For fine tuning your treatment program, *you must contact your own dermatologist!*

Let's take a woman with average skin tone through the process of learning how to use Retin-A. For illustration, we'll talk about another of my patients, Monica. Monica, 40 years old, tolerates the sun very well, being what we call a pigment type III, who sometimes burns during the first part of the season, but always ends the summer with a fairly good tan.

Type I	Always burns; never tans.
Type II	Always burns; tans very poorly.
Type III	Sometimes burns, especially at the start of the season; then tans fairly well.
Type IV	Never burns; tans very well.
Type V	Blacks.

She complains of some occasional oiliness around the "T-zone" (the forehead, nose and chin area that's shaped like a T) and rarely must she consider using a moisturizer. She has hazel eyes, brown hair and is of southern European extraction. She has minor sun damage in the form of early wrinkles obtained in her college days on the roof of her sorority building, where she spent a lot of sun time in the summer, much to the detriment of her formerly lovely skin.

Starting Retin-A for Monica is easy, if she understands the process and uses the medicine sparingly at the outset. We'll start with our standby, the new low-strength *cream* (note: the gel and liquid formulations of Retin-A are *much*

Table 1 Summary of Retin-A Dosage Forms

Strength ranking*	Dosage form	Concen-tration	Color of container	Use in radiaging
6	cream	0.025%	gray & white	The safest and usual *first* choice. Easily tolerated by almost all patients. Can be diluted (see text for directions) to make even milder.
5	cream	0.05%	blue & white	Most patients progress to this as their second agent, after adapting to the lowest-strength cream.
4	cream	0.1%	red & white	Used as third agent in the sequence, if other creams adapted to readily.
3	gel	0.01%	green & white	Used as second drug in patients with excessively oily skin. Probably about equal in strength for most patients to 0.1% cream. Not easily used under cosmetics. Women must generally use this formulation at night only.
2	gel	0.025%	orange & white	Only in the oiliest patients. Cannot easily be used under cosmetics. Women must generally use at night only.
1	liquid	0.05%	bottle	Not used in routine treatment of radiaging—too irritating.

*Strength ranking: 1 = highest, 6 = lowest. The 0.01% gel is stronger than the 0.1% cream because the gel penetrates more deeply.

Youth Alert!

Almost all my patients start the program with the new low-strength *0.025% Retin-A cream (in the gray and white tube). This is the mildest of all Retin-A preparations. If your dermatologist or your pharmacist gives you a different form, check the prescription and get what was intended.*

more irritating and are almost never the *starting* formulations for correcting radiaging), usually a small 20-gram tube, in case she has to change to a different formulation. That way she won't be stuck with an expensive medicine she can't use.

Mild Soap and Water Is Good for You!

Each night she'll cleanse off her makeup with Dove soap and a washcloth or just her fingertips (the best and safest cleansing "gadgets" anyone ever knew anyway!), using skin-temperature water, neither too hot nor too cold. What we're trying to do with such a gentle cleansing routine is *not* irritate the skin prior to the application of the Retin-A cream. We use Dove soap because of its gentleness with frequently cleansed skin. In at least two separate clinical and investigational trials, Dove has been found to be the mildest soap in history. It's the one we dermatologists advise for eczema patients—people with the tenderest skins of all. If you can't tolerate its fragrance, try the new unscented Dove, or use Purpose soap, which was made to be used with Retin-A. Neutrogena soap is another fairly mild alternative that some patients like.

An aside about soap use on the face: I'm always amazed when I see women in my office who have never, ever used soap on their faces. To some women, who learned their cleansing routines in their teens or earlier with a large

---

Youth Alert!

The four best cleansers for women (and men) on the Retin-A program are Dove soap, Cetaphil lotion, SFC lotion, and pHresh.

---

dose of family tradition and a minuscule smidgen of logic, putting soap on the face is an anathema. This is ridiculous. The best cleanser and makeup remover for the face is soap. Period. But if you can't use Dove or Purpose on your face for any reason, at least choose a gentle, non–acne-causing routine like the following:

Get a bottle of Cetaphil Lipid-Free Skin Cleanser, a new one called SFC (Soap Free Cleanser), or one called pHresh—they are extremely gentle over-the- counter lotions available at the drugstore. These lotions are quite simple, inexpensive, and oil-free—big advantages over most cleansers for facial skin. Recently, some pretty fancy tests of irritancy were done involving the various soaps and cleansers, and Cetaphil came out at the very top, as the least irritating and the least comedogenic (acne-causing) of them all! These sophisticated tests finally proved what dermatologists had suspected all along —that when it comes to cleansing, nothing is milder than Cetaphil lotion. I highly recommend it for anyone seeking a liquid cleanser for her face.

Our patient rubs on a few drops of Cetaphil lotion or SFC *very gently* with a quick, circular motion. She'll probably note when she does this that the lotion almost sudses. That's the endpoint in the cleansing process. Now the lotion is wiped off with a white, unscented tissue, like Kleenex. Or she may rinse gently with clear, skin-temperature water if she wishes, and then pat dry very gently. That's it—she's cleansed! The so-called deep cleansing is a myth and is unnecessary.

Youth Alert!

Do not *use any kind of a scrubbing pad or sponge when you start the Retin-A program! You can cause extra irritation to the skin.*

Regardless of the type and method of cleansing a person uses, I emphasize again that it be done *gently*. Scrubbing the facial skin vigorously may be equated to constantly scraping and folding a thick piece of paper. After many folds, the skin has permanent lines in it, which won't go away no matter what you use on the face. So *gentle* is the watchword for facial skin care.

All soaps are detergents, which can damage cell membranes. They particularly attack the dead skin layer and make the skin drier. Be gentle! Try to imagine that every time you rubbed or massaged your face, you could *hear* the little dead-layer cells twist, snap, and break. The noise would be deafening! So leave your face *alone* as much as possible, and you won't break down any *more* of the epidermal tissue. Heavy rubbing could also cause dermal inflammation, which can destroy the collagen bundles.

When cleansing is completed, a very gentle rinse is indicated. This is done with clear water of moderate temperature. We don't need any shocks for the delicate facial skin now.

I might add a word about a commonly held belief that it's necessary to use a hot rinse, followed by a cold rinse "to shrink pores." Nonsense. Nothing you can think of will have *any* effect on pore size. Do you think pores have little muscles around them that shrink up in the cold? I've always marveled at that quaint little bit of pseudoscience spouted by the "cosmetic experts" and "aestheticians." Pore size is a genetic trait, and nothing you can do will help that problem—with the exception, believe it or not, of using Retin-A, because this medicine *does* seem to have a good

---

Youth Alert!

You can get too close to your skin, so that minor irregularities appear to you as disease, when in fact they are on everyone's skin. To stop these worrisome misinterpretations, throw away all your magnifying mirrors as a first step to feeling good about your skin!

---

effect of extracting retained debris in the gland openings, so that the pores are less obvious and do not cast visible shadows. Small blackheads are excavated. Also, the firmer skin produced by Retin-A prevents the pores from widening.

After cleansing, Monica will pat her skin dry and then apply her Retin-A when her face is still slightly moist. Word has gotten around that one should wait 20 minutes after washing, but this is unnecessary and complicates a person's scheduling. Occasionally, the skin stings briefly, but this is of no consequence. Simplicity is preferable. Every new qualification adds to noncompliance.

Applying Retin-A

Applying Retin-A is simple. I find that my only patients who need much help in application are the men, who aren't used to putting creams on their skin. But with a little spouse assistance, a few tries will lead to perfection.

For the average person, it'll take about three small pea-size dabs of the medicine to adequately cover the face. This holds for everyone, no matter what formulation your dermatologist has given you to begin your treatment (the exception is the patient who is suspected of having *extremely* sensitive skin, or other facial skin problems, like seborrheic dermatitis, rosacea, lupus erythematosus, or aller-

Youth Alert!

*Three small pea-size dollops are all that's needed.
This is not a treatment that requires a lot of the medicine. In fact, Retin-A works in such small amounts
that some experts think much weaker compounds
would even be effective without producing any
irritation!*

gies to certain chemicals and preservatives—if you have
any of these, be sure to warn your dermatologist!).

Monica puts one pea-size dollop of cream on the middle
of each cheek, and one in the center of her forehead. She
gets close to the mirror (but not the *magnifying* mirror)
when she begins to spread it over the skin, because there
are some areas where the application of the cream is
critical.

I'll digress here a minute, to tell you about another
patient, Emma, who called my nurse after one week on
Retin-A to demand a refill on her prescription. Right away,
I knew we had a problem, because a 20-gram tube lasts
me personally about two *months* and there was no logical
way Emma should have used her first tube yet. A tube
should last at least *one* month. I thought her dog must
have eaten it or something, until the nurse told me that
she had, in fact, used it all!

With a little questioning, we found out that she was
indeed applying way too much of the cream, but the reason was not immediately apparent, until we discovered
that Emma was applying it with a *cotton swab*! Naturally,
the swab only soaks up and wastes much of the medicine,
so I directed her to stop the swabs and use her fingers—
just as for cleansing, they're the best and gentlest of applicators anyway! When we told her this, Emma asked
whether it was safe for the fingers, and it certainly is,
unless you have a disease of the skin of the hands, like
hand eczema or psoriasis. In these two cases, or if you

Youth Alert!

Don't exceed the amount of Retin-A you're told to apply or the frequency of application—if you do, excessive irritation is almost guaranteed. And remember, the best applicator is your fingers.

have any other disease of the skin, naturally you'll have to consult your dermatologist.

Amazingly, one of my patients told me she had heard (on another erroneous news report) that the medicine was to be applied only to wrinkles and only with a toothpick! That's cheating yourself out of the wonderful total face benefits of Retin-A, like buying life insurance that covers you only in the event a safe falls on you on a Thursday morning! Sure, it could happen, but why not get total coverage? Same with Retin-A. It's designed to be used over *all* radiaged skin.

Now, back to Monica. We left her right up close to the mirror, with the dollops of Retin-A on her face. She'll spread the cream slowly and gently in an ever-widening circle, starting on the forehead and proceeding with that dollop right up to and into the hairline (men who are balding should put the medicine all over their hair-thinned scalps, because these are areas of frequent and severe sun damage). She slowly and gently takes the cream right down into the eyebrow (you'd be surprised at how many premalignant sunspots I find and treat in this location!).

Youth Alert!

If you are using Retin-A on your face, remember it's for all of your face, not just certain spots, or just for wrinkles that are obvious.

=== *Youth Alert!* ===
Make sure you don't have too much Retin-A on the fingers when you apply it. That way, you won't oversmear it into and onto the lower lid areas. A good way to do this is to use the dollop on the cheeks as sort of a reservoir, from which you spread small bits of the cream ever closer to the eye socket area.

Retin-A and the Eyes

Monica must be careful around the eyes, because of the hazard of stinging when the medicine gets *into* the eyes, as well as the irritation of the gentle-skinned lids. Swelling and redness are the most common side effects in this area; stinging and burning can also result. The lids, too, gradually accommodate Retin-A; swelling means that too much has been applied. Everyone can learn to apply a very thin layer cautiously right up to the edge of the lids. Stinging will be temporary and a small price to pay for erasure of these ugly wrinkles. No real harm will occur if Retin-A is actually put into the eye. Indeed, some ophthalmologists are *treating* dry eye syndrome with Retin-A. So work it gently and thinly right up to the edges of the lids.

One word about contact lenses and Retin-A: Don't mix the two. Take your lenses out after washing your face and hands; then apply your Retin-A; then rinse off your hands before retiring.

Now Monica spreads the Retin-A all over her cheeks and especially the temples, where most of the early age lines occur. The temples seem in my experience to be especially resistant to the effects of the medicine, so don't be afraid to treat these relatively early-wrinkling areas with a good dose.

Interestingly, Retin-A is about the only thing one can use in this especially delicate area to smooth out the wrinkles here. Collagen (Zyderm) injections, which we'll talk about in Chapter 9, often bead and lump up in this area, in contrast with the nice results Zyderm usually gets elsewhere on the face.

Monica will now gently rub in any areas of the cream-colored Retin-A that are still visible. And even if you forget to gently rub in a spot or two, the cream disappears into the skin nicely anyway in just a few minutes.

Some Nonfacial Areas Need Retin-A

You may think Monica has finished applying her Retin-A for the night. Not so. Several more areas are absolutely crucial to treat. Treating them will increase her medication expense by a few cents a day, but in the long run, it'll be well worth it.

For the next area, she applies another pea-sized dollop to the V of the chest. This is the area, running from mid-collarbone to the cleavage of the breasts, and back up to the other collarbone, which sun *does* hit, and very viciously, because of our habit of tanning these areas so heavily. It's an area that frequently shows the ugly dark brown freckles and "cigarette paper" wrinkling of radiaging, especially in fair-skinned people who freckle easily. And until Retin-A came along, we could do little except a little cryosurgery for the darkest of the sun freckles that appeared.

Remember, apply Retin-A thinly to the *chest*, not to the front of the neck or underside of the chin. If you use Retin-A on the light-shaded areas of the neck, you'll almost certainly get irritation. Besides, this area doesn't really *need* Retin-A.

The four remaining areas Monica treats are the backs of the fingers, hands, wrists, and lower arms. For most patients, the same-size dollop used on the face can be used on the hands, one on each side. The bend of the elbow is *very* sensitive, and should *not* be treated. The same goes for the earlobes, which often redden from the irritation

Youth Alert!

Avoid light-shaded areas of the skin, or treat them very sparingly, because Retin-A is much more irritating on these tender-skinned areas, which haven't been damaged by sun exposure.

of the medicine. With the skim of Retin-A that remains on her fingers, she treats the back of the neck, since she's always had short hair, and sun has affected this area. Men especially should carefully treat this area. Women who have not had very short hair may not have to use Retin-A here.

The backs of the hands and forearms are important areas to treat because these are the areas that reveal a person's age most accurately, even to the carnival expert who guesses ages. Investing in an extra blip of Retin-A for these areas each night may prevent the earliest sign of old age for most people: thinning and atrophy of this skin. Retin-A also helps bleach brown age spots, often called liver spots. After many months the spots often fade into insignificance. Big age spots might benefit from a small dab of Retin-A in the morning. For many of us, it's worth a drop or two of medicine to try to prevent a case of "hideous hands" as the years pass. The problem is that most physicians and even *dermatologists* don't think about applying it here, until it's too late.

Of course, to be frank, it'll be years before we can see whether the hands will, in fact, look much better. But the medicine cannot harm skin. We know it thickens the dermis. Preliminary evidence suggests that vigorous use of Retin-A noticeably improves the back of the hands. So why wait for the years to damage your hands? Might as well start treating them now.

Monica rubs in the Retin-A gently to the backs of the hands and the fingers, right up to the mid-arms. When I started doing this to my own arms, they got fairly dry, and the mid-lower arms itched a little for the first few weeks until I adapted to the drug. In fact, for a few weeks there was a low-grade, dry, eczema-type rash there, which, unless I used my moisturizer heavily, was quite bothersome.

But Monica does carefully apply it all over the tops of the hands and fingers, where wrinkling of loose skin and premalignant sunspots can be seen quite often.

Another special word about the hands. It will take many months for the medicine to work in this area—much longer than on the face—because the hands' skin tends to be naturally thicker, and almost no one thinks to treat these areas with sunscreen or protect them from the sun. So be patient; the wrinkles, sunspots, and nasty pigment blotches took years to make—there's just nothing that will *erase* them "the day before yesterday."

Retin-A and Fingernails

Many of my patients have asked whether Retin-A will help or hurt the fingernails if it accidentally gets on them. Retin-A will not hurt the fingernails, but it's reported that it will occasionally remove fingernail polish, so you may want to be a little careful about this while applying the medicine, especially to the backs of the hands and the fingers. Will it *help* nails? Nobody knows the answer to that very interesting question, but based on its generally recognized effect of thinning out the dead layer of the skin, and considering that nails are modified keratin just like that dead skin layer, one could predict it would not make them any stronger. But the studies are just not in to be sure. However, some dermatologists have noted improvement of nail *splitting* in older persons when Retin-A is applied around the nail folds and the cuticle. This is worth a try.

Youth Alert!

Are you a redneck? Large, triangular, muddy red patches at the sides of the neck are nature's way of telling you you've gotten too much sun, or that the sun is reacting to a perfume or cosmetic in the area!

Another Strange Condition to Watch For

I should say a word here about a strange condition that many sun-damaged women (and many men, too) have, called poikiloderma (po-EE-kee-lo-der-ma) of Civatte (see-VOT). This condition (which means alternating thickened and thinned skin with variability of skin colors), discovered and described by a dermatologist named Civatte, occurs on the sides of women's necks, right in the two-by-four-inch triangles where sunlight strikes the neck. It's a sharply cut-off area of extra redness, and sometimes has a knobby-white look within the reddish-brown skin in the area. Sometimes, if you look extra closely, you can see fine, dilated, reddish blood vessels in this area, which often accompany the condition. Poikiloderma of Civatte wraps around toward the back of the neck, where it usually blends off into the surrounding skin.

This is a sign of chronic and long-standing sun damage to the sides of the neck. It's the same condition from which the term *redneck* came. Southern farmers acquired that nickname when people noticed that many of them had red necks—skin changes consistent with poikiloderma of Civatte! When you see how very dark this reaction can be in some people, you'll start to spot poikiloderma in dozens of people just walking down the street.

This rash can also be a sign of chronic photodermatitis, a pigment staining caused by wearing certain perfumes, such as Shalimar, in the light-exposed neck area, which contain substances that readily react to light, producing

> === *Youth Alert!* ===
>
> *Got some Retin-A left on your palms after your nightly application? Rub it on the back of your neck!*

an irritation resulting in a color change. My chief of dermatology used to tell women that he could *cure* the Shalimar rash—all they had to do was to hand over their bottle of the perfume. At megabucks per ounce, he never got any takers, and I suspect that more than one woman chose to ignore her rash for the fragrance (a pity, since perfume allergies are easily avoided by just applying the fragrance to the *hair* instead of the skin).

It's true that in some women poikiloderma is permanent, but in most, I've found Retin-A to help lighten the spots, especially with regular use over months to years, and especially in those with more of the tannish, muddy color rather than the reddish, predominantly blood-vessel- enlargement-type cases. Women have remarked many times since I started treating them with Retin-A for radiaging that they have indeed seen these ugly spots lighten. But since the poikiloderma is already red skin, anyone with this problem will have to be supercautious using Retin-A in this area. Any irritation at all would be a sign to temporarily stop the treatment and seek some more advice from a dermatologist.

Getting back to Monica, she has finished applying her Retin-A for the evening. She's careful *not* to apply any other creams or moisturizers over it. It's best not to have any other chemicals on the skin to interfere with Retin-A. Now she's all ready to slip into bed and let the cream work its magic all through the night. Remember, too, not to wash your face *after* applying the Retin-A! This has actually happened in my practice.

If this routine seems tedious, just remember that the more often you do it, the simpler it will get. It's quite

---

Youth Alert!

Retin-A is the only thing to be applied to the skin at bedtime. Other creams, lotions and chemicals could interfere with its action or possibly cause a greater reaction than with Retin-A alone.

---

easy—just a matter of habit, really. But you might as well get right into it, because if you actually start this program, you'll be doing this for the rest of your life.

The next morning, Monica awakens and begins a simple routine before applying her cosmetics. All she need do is wash her face (if she wants to—it's not mandatory) and apply a heavy moisturizer. Sounds too easy to be true, doesn't it? The third most crucial part of the Retin-A program, after the drug itself, naturally, and a sunscreen, is the morning moisturizer. Why? Because after almost two years of using Retin-A personally, I *still* have mild scaling of my facial skin, and so do many of my patients. But you can see the scaliness vanish instantly when you apply a safe and gentle moisturizer. A great sunscreen like Solbar 50 often functions as a wonderful moisturizer by itself, so an extra moisturizer may not be necessary.

The World's Best Moisturizers

That brings up the whole subject of the "right" moisturizer to use with Retin-A. There is certainly no lack of choices. The ones I recommend are excellent, tried-and-proven softening lotions and creams I've tested personally and on my patients for use with the Retin-A program. This is not to say there aren't others that will work too, but these are the ones *I* use on my own skin and advise my patients to use.

Johnson & Johnson, the parent company that manufactures Retin-A, recommends Purpose cream, which for months was the only one I recommended. But after a few months of advising Retin-A patients to use it, I had an occasional complaint of stinging. It *did*, in fact, seem to be a great moisturizer, but the occasional stinging in some patients was bothersome. Most of the women who complained of this learned to live with it.

So far, the best and *least* stinging ones that still do an efficient job of moisturizing are Complex-15 *cream* (Schering Co.)and Moisturel *cream* (Westwood). Both can be bought in drugstores, over the counter (no prescription required). Both of these creams are available in lotions, too, but the creams are more moisturizing.

Other moisturizers my patients have had success with while on Retin-A are Eucerin lotion, and a really heavy one that feels like Crisco (but some patients need just that to stay moist), Eucerin cream. Just remember to apply any moisturizer you use very thinly—you still have to put on a sunscreen (most mornings) and then your cosmetics!

Monica has washed gently this morning with Dove, patted dry with a soft, absorbent towel, and has applied a thin layer of moisturizer. What should she do now? Apply *another* thin layer, following what I call the "Bark Double Layer Moisturization Technique." All my years in dermatology have convinced me that this is the most efficient way to guarantee that dry, Retin-A-treated skin will stay soft and supple.

One more word about moisturizers: the best ones are *not* expensive. The more expensive ones (I've seen them up to $60-$70 per *ounce*!) just have more chemicals added that you do not need. No use adding any problems, like topical allergies, to your Retin-A regimen.

Sunscreens and Retin-A

Moisturizing is vital to keep the side effects of Retin-A treatment from showing every day, but using the proper

Youth Alert!

Don't even consider trying the Retin-A program
unless you're willing to do two things:
  1. Swear off intentional tanning exposure.
  2. Use the highest-rated sunscreen you can get
your hands on whenever there's a risk of sun
exposure.

sunscreens is the single most important step in *preventing*
more damage to Monica's soon-to-be-beautiful-again skin.

Sunscreens are a marvelous invention. Think of it! By
designing and mixing just the right chemicals, it's possible to give nearly complete protection to sun-exposed skin.
Here's how the SPF ("sun protection factor") system works:

Say you ordinarily get a slight sunburn after about 30
minutes in the sun. With an SPF 10 sunscreen, you would
theoretically be able to remain in the same sunlight for
300 minutes (5 hours) before getting the same burn!

For years we had only the low-numbered sunscreens,
like SPF 8 and SPF 10. Then dermatologic chemistry
advanced into the SPF 15 sunscreens, which were a significant and wonderful advance in protection. Many of
these sunscreens contained PABA (para-aminobenzoic
acid), an efficient sunscreen but occasionally an irritating
one, too.

The photobiology experts say that if children were to
use only the second-generation 15-rated sunscreens from
ages 1–18, they would happily *avoid* 78% of the effects of
all the wrinkle-causing and cancer-causing radiation they
would ever be exposed to. What I'm telling you is that
using a powerful sunscreen on your children should be
ranked right up there with giving love and providing a
good education!

But now we can do even *better*. We're now into the third-
generation sunscreens, which will protect a person up to
30–50 times as long as he could ordinarily stay out in the

Youth Alert!

Want to do your children a favor that could possibly keep their skin healthy and looking good for a life-time? Use at least a 15-rated sunscreen on them during every sun exposure from age 1-18, and encourage them to get into the habit of using sunscreens for a lifetime! Just think, doing this may even eliminate the need for a Retin-A program in the future!

sun before burning. The best of these advanced screens, or as I call them, "parasols in a bottle," are Presun 29 (Westwood), four ounces for $6.50, Sundown 30 (Johnson & Johnson), four ounces for $8.50, and one more amazing one I'll tell you about shortly. Each is available over the counter. Some of these wonderful advances in sun management do not even contain PABA, and are waterproof for up to two 40-minute swims, making them the first ones that can be talked about as all-day sunscreens. In fact, they're so strong you may not need to reapply them during a whole day's outing. Still, I tell my patients to reapply them if they will be out a long time or swimming for very extended periods. The newest Presun, called Presun 39 (four ounces for $7), does contain PABA, and is waterproof. If you're not PABA-sensitive, it's a really astounding protection for sun-sensitive, Retin-A–treated skin.

Several other sunscreens deserve mention for their high sun protection factors and their relative nonirritancy of the skin in Retin-A–treated patients. One is Elizabeth Arden's Sun Science, an SPF 34 sunscreen that usually will not cause any stinging in Retin-A patients. And patients tell me it's a lot less greasy-feeling, too. Remember, though, that it has a PABA derivative in it, just in case you have an allergy to that chemical. Cost? About $12.50 for 3-1/2 ounces, and well worth it.

Presun 15 For Faces (Westwood) is almost completely nonirritating to facial skin, but needs to be reapplied after swimming. It's about $6.50 for a four-ounce tube.

One other lotion deserves special mention: Solbar PF (2½ ounces for $6). The "PF" stands for "PABA-free," and I've never heard of this sunscreen irritating a face. But it, too, demands reapplication after water exposure. And it has an SPF of only 15.

A new, almost unbelievable advance in sunscreens was recently introduced, Solbar PF Ultra *50*, which has the highest SPF I've ever heard of. Wearing this sunscreen is like standing in a dark basement at midnight! It costs around $8.00 for four ounces.

One more item about sunscreens: Just because I've said not to apply Retin-A to the front of the neck and to use it only sparingly on the eyelids, that does *not* mean you should withhold your *sunscreen* in these areas! You *must* use a terrific sunscreen everywhere, especially if you are really interested in pursuing a "youth miracle" for your skin. And while on the general subject of sunscreens, make sure you use only a cosmetic system that contains a sunscreen. Many of the lines I'll mention in Chapter 5 do contain mild- to moderate-rated sunscreens.

Retin-A and Your Skin Tone

Monica has medium-toned skin and thus can probably tolerate the undiluted low-strength Retin-A cream, but many women who are of Scotch-Irish and Nordic descent, or other such light-skinned types, may not tolerate its use nightly, even in the newly released lowest strength. Does that mean they will not get an effect from their use of Retin-A cream? Not at all—Retin-A experts believe that the cream works in minuscule amounts, like 0.001%! In fact, some clinicians have gone so far as to ask Johnson & Jonson (Retin-A's manufacturer) to formulate a new, lower strength, but so far no moves have been taken outside of

=== *Youth Alert!* ===

The lighter-skinned you are, the more caution you must exercise in starting Retin-A. Dilution of even the low-strength cream is often necessary!

the recent release of the new 0.025% cream. Representatives of the company described how difficult it is to make any changes in their formulations, in view of strict FDA regulations. They had to go through a whole new series of difficult stability tests for the drug just to change the *tube size*, without even changing the drug one iota! These special tubes are even Teflon-coated to prevent waste.

But strength of the medicine is certainly important. Take my patient Shawn. She's a fair-skinned, 28-year-old, freckly redhead of Scotch-Irish descent. She has a chronic problem with dry skin (she says her skin feels like "scaly leather" when it gets dry) and needs constant moisturization for her face, especially during the winter.

She's a person who has always loved the sun and actually does pursue a tan, even though the "tan" she develops never gets anywhere near tan or brown in color and is always preceded by a blistering burn. Her skin after sunlight exposure could be described as a muddy beige, with a few greenish freckles thrown in for good measure. In short, her skin, because of its genetics, never learned to tan and is completely untrainable in this regard. All she'd get by sunbathing would be further precancerous changes, wrinkles, laxity, abnormal pigmentation or colored spots, and a burned-out, muddy, blemished, aged look. She has Type I skin.

Maybe you're thinking that pale-skinned, sensitive Shawn would never be a good candidate for Retin-A? Not at all. In this instance, we use the lowest-strength cream (gray and white tube) and ask the pharmacist to dilute it with an equal amount of Moisturel cream, or Purpose cream.

That cuts down the power and irritancy of the medicine and adds a moisturizer to help with the dryness that accompanies the treatment.

In some patients, I've actually cut the strength of the Retin-A down to one-fourth of the original strength. For most light-skinned patients this lower concentration will work, although even at the diluted strength some will have minor irritation, dryness, and flaking. You should know that, although this works well in *my* patients, Dr. Kligman will not use this formulation, saying it has not been proven to be stable. Instead, he uses alternate-night treatments.

What if you have skin like Shawn's? Since some physicians will not be accustomed to prescribing Retin-A for use in radiaging, here is that prescription exactly as it is written in English on the prescription pad, so that you can just take this book with you to the dermatologist's office and *show* it to him:

For the half-strength cream:

Pharmacist: mix well the following:

Retin-A cream, 0.025%, 20 grams

Moisturel cream, 20 grams

Sig: Apply thinly as directed to facial, arm and hand areas every other night or less to start.

And for the one-fourth-strength mixture:

Pharmacist: mix well the following:

Retin-A cream, 0.025%, 20 grams

Moisturel cream, 60 grams

Sig: Apply thinly as directed to facial, arm and hand areas every other night or less to start.

Everything else in Shawn's regimen is the same as the darker-skinned Monica's, except that Shawn will have to cleanse even more gently and moisturize more frequently and heavily. And side effects will begin to appear more

---

Important!

Having access to the above prescriptions and, in fact, to this book should not lead you to ask your "friendly pharmacist" for this medicine, or even your friendly family practitioner for a prescription, just because you supposedly now know how to use it. Lack of dermatologic care and guidance is the chief reason people fail to remain on the program.

---

quickly with Shawn's treatment than with Monica's. Let's talk about some of them.

Side Effects

Keep in mind that we've been using this medicine for 18 years in some patients without stopping—they are the ones who alerted us to its effect in radiaging!—so the possibility of there being long-term side effects that no one knows about yet is dimming with each passing year. But still, almost every day in my practice I hear patients say (usually because someone with the wrong information has scared the hell out of them), "Oh, I'd better not try that stuff until it gets a few years of thorough testing under its belt!" It brings up our family's favorite saying, "A mind changed against its will is of the same opinion still!" After years of dealing with the pseudoscience expounded in the lay press, over the back fence with the neighbors, and in the media, I'm used to accepting the truth of that old saw.

You already know about some of the side effects of Retin-A—drying and irritation. But what you need to know now is the course of events that follows the first few days of Retin-A use on facial skin.

In the first few days, some patients have noted some tenderness. This is most noticeable around the corners of the nose, where the wings of the nose attach to the cheeks, but it can also be noticed near the lids, the corners of the mouth, and under the chin. Keep in mind that a little redness, the "rosy glow" of Retin-A users, is to be expected as the medicine dilates, or opens up, many of the superficial blood vessels and later generates new ones. In the older age group in whom the superficial blood vessels have been wiped out by chronic sun damage, Retin-A induces new blood vessel growth, causing some of the rosy glow, too. This redness, or pinkness, really, is *not* an allergy, but just a mild irritation, which will fade with continuous use.

Flaking is another nuisance problem, which almost always accompanies dryness from the medicine. I've been using the drug for a couple of years now, and I *still* have a mild, noninflammatory flaking. However, there was some true inflammation (redness and soreness) of my face at the outset of the treatment. When I began to teach women how to apply this medicine and what to expect, I'd often go into the office in the morning without having applied the very moisturizer I instructed *them* to use, just so I could demonstrate to new Retin-A patients just exactly what the flaking looked like! I wised up quickly, and started showing the patients pictures and slides instead. Now *I'm* much more comfortable, too, as are my patients.

From three to five weeks into the treatment process, you'll possibly notice some small reddish patches coming out. These are usually flat but very slightly rough to the touch when you run your finger over them. These are little actinic keratoses (AKs) which are premalignant sunspots. If they are already in your skin, they will pop out and be destroyed by Retin-A as you continue to apply it. These should not be misunderstood as irritation spots.

One patient of mine was greatly alarmed when she saw isolated red spots appearing on her face several weeks into the treatment. She was *sure* she had developed an allergy to the medicine and made a special urgent appointment to see me three weeks into her treatment so I could evaluate them. They were AKs, all right. Naturally, all she needed was a little reassurance. That accom-

$$=== \textit{Youth Alert!} ===$$

Watch for your Retin-A "merit badges"—the little red, scaly spots that indicate the medicine is wiping out true troublemakers, which would have been skin cancers later!

plished, I sent her on her way till her routine two-month follow-up.

Another thing you'll notice with advancing weeks after beginning Retin-A is exceptional facial smoothness. Most people describe it as a wonderful and youthful softness and suppleness to the skin, which really does remind me of the smooth softness of a baby's bottom. The explanation for this probably has to do with the thinning of the skin's dead layer, which when thick adds stiffness and brittleness to the skin, as in the elderly who have had a lot of sun damage and naturally dry skin.

Everybody seems to like this "side effect," but it does also indicate a certain sensitivity in the skin, which should warn you to avoid harsh chemicals and further sun damage. This is your skin in its most beautiful, naked state, and it requires special care.

Retin-A Faces Are Tender Places!

Want to know just how tender your skin can get? Another friend and patient named Pat came in one day with large, weeping sore spots on her face. Pat had been on Retin-A for four weeks and had just come into my office from the beauty shop, where she had gotten her usual monthly waxing treatment for facial hair. All went well, she thought, as the cosmetician applied the same wax at the same temperature she had used on Pat's face for years, but on removing the hair, the wax also removed what little dead

```
================= Youth Alert! =================

  Don't have any facial treatments, such as waxing,
  while using Retin-A, without the approval of your
  dermatologist. To do so may be courting disaster!
  Talk to your dermatologist about everything you do
  to your skin, such as toners, astringents, scrubbers,
  tan-in-a-bottle.
```

layer was left after her four weeks of continuous nightly Retin-A treatment! It was a consequence that neither patient nor beautician could have anticipated. The lesson to be learned here: Retin-A patients should ask the dermatologist *first*, before getting *anything* done to areas involved in Retin-A treatment. I would have suggested, even though I had not heard of that particular complication before, that they test a tiny area at the edge of the face before doing the entire cheeks. A simple phone call might have saved Pat some pain, misery, and worry about her face. You should know, however, that Pat healed excellently, and in just a few short weeks she looked better and more beautiful than ever.

Controlling Retin-A–Induced Acne Bumps

If you're acne-prone, you may have a few unpleasant side effects in store for you when you start on Retin-A. Even though the drug was designed and approved initially for the *treatment* of acne, clinicians found that the drug actually *aggravated* acne and produced new bumps before the disease began to clear. This has been a constant source of consternation to my patients whenever I've started them on Retin-A for treatment of acne. In my experience, Retin-A seems to project pre-existing acne bumps to the surface of the skin, where they seem to resolve quickly.

=== *Youth Alert!* ===

*The best acne suppressant while starting on Retin-A
(if you're indeed even acne prone) is tetracycline.
Hazards and warnings? The major ones are sun sensitivity and stomach irritation. And remember, tetracycline is not permitted under the age of eight, nor
while a woman is pregnant.*

This whole acne exacerbation process can take 2 to 12
weeks, much the same as with initiation of a course of
Accutane, where lesions also get worse before they get
better. Often, I put the patients with significant acne flares
on internal antibiotics while they are trying to adapt to
the topical Retin-A. This helps prevent the new bumps,
as they begin the medicine designed to eventually control
their pimples *and* help reverse some of the ravages of sun
and time. Dermatologists hate to have to cause a new
problem while getting rid of one, but sometimes that's
necessary on at least a very temporary basis.

The best of the oral antibiotics for acne is oral tetracycline, which has been used very safely for acne suppres-
sion for many, many years. It is my choice for the usual
patient starting out on Retin-A, if he or she has a problem
with new bumps arising. I find this to be a special problem for women around the time of menstrual periods,
because of the generally recognized worsening of acne
then.

Topical antibiotics and lotions like the ones we use in
greasy teenagers are usually too strong and irritating to
be used in the acne flare that accompanies the first few
weeks of Retin-A therapy. In general, if you try to use them
you'll get too dry, and have a lot more stinging and irritation than the usual Retin-A patient.

Here's a minor but chancy point to consider: A certain
small percentage of people on tetracycline who expose
themselves to even minimal amounts of sunlight get a

photodermatitis that looks like a fiery red sunburn. If this same person happened to be using Retin-A simultaneously, the reaction might be extremely severe. I have not seen this yet, but I'm waiting. And I take special precautions to warn my patients about this very distressing possibility. This gives the dermatologist a second very valid reason to elicit the "Retin-A Pledge" not to engage in intentional sun exposure! If you consider that I also use a lot of Retin-A in my acne-patient population, and I have not yet seen this combination of complications, it must be extraordinarily rare. Still, to be forewarned is to be forearmed. Consider yourself forewarned, and avoid sun if you're on both drugs.

One more "side effect" to remember about Retin-A, if you get up to the gel strengths: The gels are in a liquid that contains a cellulose mixture which, if applied too heavily, can ball up when you apply your cosmetics. This phenomenon is called "pilling." The secret here is to apply the medicine very, very thinly, even though intuitively you'd think that anything starting out that thinly probably couldn't do any real good. You're wrong, as you'll appreciate if you ever work up to starting these higher-strength gel formulations. Let's talk about some of them.

Stronger Formulations

We've talked about the low-strength Retin-A cream forms (0.025% and 0.05% concentrations), but there are several stronger formulations that you may see and hear about from time to time, shown in Table 1.

Some people desire a little quicker dryness because they ordinarily have oilier complexions; for them, increasing the strength makes good sense. Also, some people just aren't comfortable using a medicine unless they can actually *see* an effect, such as dryness and flakiness, and if these signs disappear as the patients accommodate to the Retin-A, they may need a stronger strength to "keep

Youth Alert!

*In order of increasing strength of Retin-A, the prepa-
rations go like this: 0.025% cream, 0.05% cream,
0.1% cream, 0.01% gel, 0.025% gel, and 0.5% liquid.
Some dermatologists would maintain that the 0.01%
gel is equal in strength to the 0.1% cream.*

them going," psychologically, that is. These are people who
demand a lot from themselves and their medicine, including visible signs that "something's actually happening."

The liquid form of Retin-A is the most powerful of all
and is not used in my program, because of irritation.

Recapping all these dosages and formulations reminds
me again of Jenny, who we discussed at the start of this
chapter, and who got her prescription for high-strength
Retin-A gel from her cardiologist neighbor. When the news
of Retin-A's reversal of radiaging first broke, people all
over the country were rushing to buy any form of it they
could find, just to get some of the "magic medicine."

People pursuing a nicer-looking skin can be very, very
persistent. The rush was on for Retin-A, as proved by the
response to the first Retin-A seminar we held in the office
for people who wanted to learn how to use it. There was
literally no Retin-A to be found anywhere in the country—not for acne patients nor for radiaging patients. Many
of those people who ran out and bought up all that tretinoin are no longer using Retin-A because of the irritation
these stronger forms caused, and because they completely
lacked directions such as this chapter to tell them what
to expect.

Bottom line? Retin-A is a powerful medicine with side
effects, just as other medicines have side effects. There is
no *perfect* medicine, without side effects and with a perfect safety record. But with the help of your dermatologist
and this book, you can lower the risk of negative side
effects.

5

Cosmetics and Retin-A

No one dies of old skin.
—Albert M. Kligman, MD

Cosmetics can be a real bugaboo not only for Retin-A patients but even for nonusers, because of the frequent and often unidentified irritation of the skin they cause, and, on occasion, allergy to them. In fact, when I first started my practice, I was taught that women patients, especially women acne patients, really shouldn't wear *any* cosmetics, because they cause so many problems. However, in the first few months I found that proscription utterly ridiculous. Often, I'd see the same women I had just admonished for wearing heavy layers of cosmetics reapplying their foundation on the way out of my office to their cars! It was a completely impractical ban for our modern, beauty-oriented age, and I soon realized that.

How to Find the Right Cosmetics

There's no way a woman can adequately analyze the thousands of cosmetic formulations available to her to see which is the safest. The way to pick a cosmetic, or in fact a whole line of cosmetics, is to ask the advice of a dermatologist. There are several companies that make very safe cosmetics and cooperate excellently with dermatologists in studying irritation, allergy, and most important, what we

---

Youth Alert!

In my experience, the least troublesome cosmetic lines for Retin-A patients are Dermage, Clinique, Allercreme, and Dermablend.

---

call acnegenesis—the ability of a product or even a whole cosmetic line to cause or worsen acne.

The four companies I'll mention are ones whose products have ultra-low incidence of irritation, cosmetic allergies, and aggravation of acne, and with which I've had considerable success in sensitive, acne-prone patients over the past 15 years. And while acne doesn't have a whole lot to do with the wrinkling phenomenon of radiaging, I would advise *anyone*, on the Retin-A program or not, to give her skin its best chance by using the best types of cosmetics. If you figured out how many pounds of cosmetics a woman uses during her lifetime, you'd understand the need for the mildest of ingredients and totally tested cosmetic systems.

The product lines I heartily and actively recommend are:

Dermage. This company produces a beautifully non-acne-causing line of cosmetics incorporating the simple principle that, with time, the skin varies in its moisture content. Therefore, they have two different lines of cosmetic formulations—the "Mauve" line for teens with an oil-related problem, like acne, whiteheads, and blackheads, and the "Pearl" line for women with slightly dry skin.

Of course, the Pearl line is the one I'd generally recommend for patients on the Retin-A program, because of its softening properties. It's like a moisturizer, sunscreen, and a cosmetic all rolled into a single formulation. Generally, women with the drying induced by Retin-A do much better on this brand of makeup.

The Dermage line has two important "inconveniences." The first is that it is made by and for dermatologists, and therefore is generally available only in their offices. The reason for the exclusivity is that this is a really different cosmetic system, and users need to get instructions on its special method of application before jumping into the program. It's not quite as easy a system to apply, but it's supersafe, and I can't give any system a higher recommendation.

The second "disadvantage" is that the company does not as yet make eye makeup, except mascara. This is unfortunate, because many dermatologists would love to have a system for the eye areas that is as safe for sensitive patients as the general Dermage system. If you'd like to find a dermatologist in your area who can teach you about Dermage, call 800-334-8173.

Clinique. This company has produced, in my experience, the most consistently fine, fragrance-free over-the-counter line of cosmetics in the history of dermatology. They are widely available at better stores. It could be said that Clinique is the standard recommendation of dermatologists treating allergy-prone and acne-prone patients.

Faults in the Clinique line? While they're few and far between, I can say that their salespeople (always busily running around in white lab coats) *look* a lot more competent in skin care than they really are. But if you take the system for what it's worth—that is, a good and safe cosmetic product—you'll probably be safe and secure in the use of at least part of their system.

One caution: While on the Retin-A program, you should be using only their *makeup*—that is, only the foundation (Pore Minimizer and the other Clinique foundations are OK), powder blush, and any of their eye cosmetics you'd like. You should still follow *my* recommendations regarding cleansing and should not let yourself be talked into using their soaps, astringents, scrubs, or any other facial products, unless you get direct orders to do so from your own dermatologist. Also, don't even consider having your face "analyzed" by their "oil computer" gadget while you're using Retin-A. Their people may not understand anywhere as much as you do about Retin-A. Ask your dermatologist about your skin type—he is a much better source of information. Want to find a local retailer handling Clinique? Call 212-572-4458.

Allercreme. This amazing little company, which has been around since my beginnings in dermatology, has consistently supported the pursuit of cosmetic excellence. In fact, besides carefully communicating to dermatologists exactly what ingredients are contained *in* their lines, Allercreme has gone the extra mile by actually (on occasion) developing *individual* cosmetics for women who show an allergy to one or more of their products! Now, that's the kind of service that's as rare as a spare tube of Retin-A!

Seriously, it is a superb line of cosmetics for use with my program. Try them. The line is usually available in pharmacies, and you can usually find a supplier by talking to your own dermatologist. If you cannot, call 817-293-0450 and ask for local distributors information.

Dermablend. This is a relatively new addition to the specialty dermatological-type cosmetics, for which the reports from my fellow dermatologists are especially good. Because of those favorable reports, I would approve them for use with Retin-A. Their number is 201-905-5200.

The Bottom Line on Cosmetics

It all comes down to this. The use of Retin-A on a woman's face is not an easy program to go through. Irritation results from the medicine alone, and that's why it's necessary not to fan the fires with any other irritants. You'll be tempted to take the word of cosmetic companies that their cosmetics are approved for use with my program, but don't you believe it. You've seen what I recommend for my patients in my own office, and recommendations outside

of these are extremely unusual. Don't even consider anything else, even if you've been using a cosmetic system for
years, unless you're willing to gamble on some pretty severe
irritation of your tender skin.

A special note should be added here about rip-off cosmetics and cosmetic systems that are trying to cash in on
the positive Retin-A research findings. First, you should
realize that Retin-A is *not* found in any cosmetic systems
or formulations. Period. It simply is *not* available for over-
the-counter use in *anything*! No other substance is available *anywhere* with the properties of Retin-A, with the
possible exception of alpha-hydroxy acids, such as lactic
acid and glycolic acid. Recent tests indicate that these
preparations are showing mild signs of aiding in the anti-
wrinkle fight.

Why Retin-A Won't Go Over the Counter

Retin-A is *not* FDA-approved for use in pregnancy and
may never be. The reasons for this are several: We know
that retinoids (the vitamin A class of drugs as a whole)
taken orally are teratogenic (cause fetal organs not to form
correctly). While no one to my knowledge has ever linked
fetal malformations to any topically applied preparation,
no dermatologist, and certainly no pharmaceutical company, ever wants to test *that* hypothesis (in the rat studies
in which abnormalities were reported, it was necessary
to use *50 times the amount* of Retin-A that would be used
in human skin!). So don't ever expect to see Retin-A made
an over-the-counter drug, unless some pretty detailed
research somehow proves the notion that the drug could
never cause a fetal malformation. And proving a negative
result in any series of tests is nearly impossible.

Therefore, although putting a fantastic compound like
Retin-A into cosmetics for everyday use *sounds* like the

answer, it'll never happen. Such availability would not allow for the fine tuning and adjustment of the dosage of the drug in new patients. Someday, maybe a retinoid will be developed that will not pass through the skin into the bloodstream, but as of the date of publication of this book, no such agent has been found—every chemical put on the skin has the potential to be absorbed into the blood.

This is why many dermatologists think all cosmetics should be labeled as "drugs," since they clearly affect and influence the function and sometimes the very structure of the skin, and frequently aggravate skin diseases. Labeled as such, they would have to undergo extensive testing to *prove* their claims that they could "rejuvenate" skin or make it look younger. Thankfully, the FDA has finally taken a sterner stance regarding these claims. In April 1988, the authorities issued an order to cosmetic manufacturers to stop making such unsubstantiated claims for their products, and to tone down their ads and their labels to conform with the modest properties of cosmetics as opposed to drugs.

And that's the basic reason those companies don't want to have to prove their claims: *They can't!* They don't ever want to be forced into the position of doing the tests that will make them *admit* their products are no more than fair-to-good coverups for the skin. If its product really worked to reverse aging, don't you think a company would be eager to *do* the studies necessary to demonstrate that fact in ethical dermatological journals? Of course they would. But they know they'd fail, and they could never risk it!

Keeping It Simple

Let me tell you a story about my biochemistry training in medical school. I was doing an experiment one day in which I was to make a small quantity of aspirin in the laboratory. It had to be pure, and the quantity had to be

---

Youth Alert!

Don't expect to find tretinoin in cosmetics any time soon. Side effects will prevent that. But they won't prevent cosmetic companies from making claims that they have compounds "similar" to Retin-A in their products. Save your money—you know better!

---

exact, so I went through a detailed washing recipe that involved several steps, instead of the one that was recommended to us by the professor who taught the course. At the final wash of the white, powdered aspirin, almost my entire product washed away! My lab grade that day reflected my disappointment, and I approached the biochemist to ask what I had done wrong.

"Dr. Lester," I said, with a certain disbelief in my voice, "I used the best and most detailed washing system I could for this experiment, and my product *still* disappeared! I just don't understand it."

"Bark," said the good doctor, "I'm going to give you a lesson that I hope follows you for the rest of your medical career: You can be *too* detailed sometimes. You can *overdo*, as well as underdo. Always use the K.I.S.S. method whenever possible."

"OK, I give up. What's the K.I.S.S. method?"

"Keep It Simple, Stupid!"

Youth Alert!

Keep your cosmetic routine simple. You don't need to slather on creams, lotions, or potions while you're using Retin-A. Basically, you need a good moisturizer and good, non–acne-causing, nonirritating cosmetics. Refuse any and all facials, saunas, sun treatments, and massage, because all they will do is damage your face.

Well, I've remembered that philosophy ever since, and it's helped me innumerable times. And it applies to cosmetics used with Retin-A. You don't need a lot of gunky lotions, toners, astringents, bracers, exfoliators, rejuvenators, or skin polishers when you're on Retin-A. For the most part, companies that sell you that stuff are out to do just that—*sell* the stuff. You don't have to pay a million dollars an ounce for the magical Oil of African Rhino Horn for your face. Remember, *K.I.S.S.*! Expensive doesn't mean *better*—it just means *expensive*! So save your hard-earned bucks, and buy some simple-but-good products to accompany your use of Retin-A. They'll serve you much better in the long run.

6

The Truth About Tanning Parlors

There's a sucker born every minute.
—*P.T. Barnum*

Back in the 1920s and 1930s, this country was a nation of beautiful, smooth-skinned people, conscientious about their skin health. It was referred to as the "parasol and bonnet generation," the members of which thought, for whatever reason, that a tan was undesirable. Sadly, that ethic changed in the 40s and 50s.

We dermatologists lament the passing of those highly protective "physical" sunscreens, but we welcomed the advent of sunscreens produced by modern chemistry to provide some real protection for the human skin.

The Quest for the "Great American Tan"

Where did Americans ever get the idea that a tan was to be admired rather than ashamed of? How did we turn from a country where Caucasians protected themselves from the sun to a country where the "leathery look" was in, and smooth, untanned skin was definitely out? The answer is eminently clear: leisure time and our quest for status. After World War II, people were more affluent. They began going on vacations and would come back with the Great American Tan.

So having a tan became a status symbol. Gradually, this obsession with tanning brought about shortcuts in the way of sunlamps, tanning booths, and other similar travesties. Entrepreneurs in the "tanning industry" found it profitable to entice youngsters into pursuing the darkest and most damaging tans.

The market proved phenomenal for those who put their money into production of the booths. In 1985 over 8,000 of the booths were sold in this country alone for *home* use. And at the outset, since the studies that showed all the harm they do had not yet been conducted, the manufacturers even managed to get *dermatologist* sponsors for the units, which would eventually be the benchmark around which the entire industry rotated—a virtual mask of professional respectability, from which they could spout untruths by the bucketful, convincing us and our kids that these units were safe for the darkening of human skin.

The Skin Doomsday Machine

If you were to sit down one evening with the brightest minds in our country to devise the most significant threat to human skin in the history of man, it would take you but a few minutes to conclude that that threat, if it were to maximally damage our bodies' largest organ, would have to have the following requirements:

1. *Intensity*. It should cause severe burns in some very unlucky individuals. It should be over 1,000 times more powerful than natural sunlight, which we already know can kill you, given enough exposure.

2. *Depth*. The damaging light from the units should penetrate into the deep dermis, the layer that is the most sensitive to all the types of damage discussed in this book.

3. *Kills immune cells.* To really hurt someone, the ultraviolet A rays should penetrate into the deep dermal blood vessels, where the sensitive immune cells of the body are circulating constantly.

4. *Destroys blood vessels in the skin.* This fact is discussed elsewhere in this book, but suffice it to say that the blood vessels are not only penetrated by UVA light, they are annihilated by it, slowly and progressively.

5. *Reacts with topical agents and medicines already in the body to make horrendous skin rashes.* The light, to be most discomfort-causing, should be able to react with everything from antibacterial, deodorant soaps to medicines used for diabetes, nerve and emotional disorders, high blood pressure, and many others.

6. *Causes laxity in the skin.* The skin of patients who have exposed themselves to the light you devise should look as bad as possible. And just for completeness, wouldn't it be wonderful if the color produced in the skin were an *awful* orangish/red that's spottable about a mile away in a heavy user?

7. *Causes early aging.* If you could see some of the patients who have a disease called psoriasis, you could see the progressive destruction that occurs when certain lights and certain wavelengths are used to treat it. For dermatologists, this is an unappealing treatment to have to employ to get the psoriatic patient better, but we use it only in the most severe psoriatics, who have not been helped by the many other treatments used for this problem. Most of these psoriatic patients are so miserable that the risk of a higher number of skin cancers in years to come is a mere calculated trade-off. Some of these patients, when seen initially, would have gladly jumped off a bridge rather than suffer one more night of the disease. So it's not hard to imagine why even this treatment is accepted by these patients.

But for our Skin Doomsday Machine, we couldn't ask for a better armament with which to clobber the skin.

8. *Causes skin cancers, possibly melanoma* in years to come. These are the so-called time bombs of ultraviolet exposure that won't go off for years. We've known that most types of skin cancer are caused by sunlight, and this "safe" UVA that our Doomsday Committee will design is no exception. Maybe, just maybe, if we really put our minds to the design of this thing, we could activate a whole new cohort of skin cancers in our tanning population that will come back to haunt us in the years to come. And if we *really* do our deadly business well enough, perhaps we could overwhelm the dermatologists and other surgeons who will have to take care of these tumors in the future.

9. *Causes ugly pigmentation of the skin.* Perhaps we could make this phototorture chamber reproduce the mottled skin color of the chronically sun-damaged as I once saw demonstrated to me by one of my teenage patients who was addicted to "free" tanning. She was just 17, but already had many of the brown spots of old age on her chest and arms. She was also almost covered with strange-looking brownish moles that were quite disturbing. I biopsied about 10 of these, which I thought warranted a closer look due to their clinical appearance, and each and every one of them was a premelanoma—a so-called dysplastic nevus— very dangerous lesions, to say the least. Perhaps we could get our "Skin Weapon" to make these spots on people?

10. *Transmits the herpes simplex virus (HSV) and fungal and bacterial skin diseases.* I have seen this so many times in my office that it's scary. Patients who have just started frying themselves in the tanning coffins come in a few days after contracting typical herpes simplex blisters on the *center of the back*—not by anyone's estimation a usual place for that disease to form. It *is* possible, unfortunately, to contract HSV from the wet exudate or drippings of someone else who has lain practically nude in that tanning bed just before you. Who knows what they clean those things with? Are you going to trust *your* skin to the efforts of a nonmedical or nonparamedical person, and depend

on him to rid that apparatus of all infectious diseases before *you* get in? Not me, brother.

It'll come as no surprise to anyone that this very worst threat you could possibly devise, our so-called Skin Doomsday Machine, would be the indoor tanning booth. The tanning booth would be the "perfect" destroyer of skin for these reasons and many more that are just now being discovered.

So isn't there any safe way to tan? *Absolutely not!* Remember the "dermatologist's equation," Tan = damage. If you're tanned, you're damaged.

Why, then, doesn't somebody *do* something about these units? How can our government let these things proliferate, when so many other regulations are passed to limit exposure from everything from bacteria to carcinogens? Aren't we surely doing as much damage with these units?

"Free" Country Doesn't Always Mean "Safe" Country

The problem is that in a free land, entrepreneurs can start any business they want, as long as it doesn't *obviously* hurt anybody. But the laws are much subtler concerning gradual harm that shows up in later years. These tanning machines are permanently ensconced in our society simply because it took a while for scientists to devise tests that could adequately show just how severe the damage they produce is. In other words, the entrepreneurs got there "the firstest with the mostest," just as have so many others in the past. And they certainly *do* have the dollars behind them. It's a truly massive industry—with its own trade journals masquerading under extraordinarily healthy-sounding names, with pictures of gorgeous people (by *their* standard) plastered everywhere.

And the tanning units go under the guise of "fitness" in most places, being chiefly found in hairdressers' salons and "health" clubs that profess to actually be doing their clients a service. In fact, when I joined a true health club a couple of years ago, my first question to the membership salesperson was, "Do you have any sort of tanning facilities?" I almost sprained a finger signing up when the salesperson replied, "Oh, no, we couldn't do that in good conscience—haven't you heard what those things *do* to you?"

As if we didn't have enough to deal with with the thinning of the earth's ozone layer, we now have the damage concentrated right up close to the skin, emanating from bulbs not inches away.

If your neighborhood's like mine, you can't even get an appointment for these things. People (most of them kids who claim not to know any better) are lined up out into the street to get into them, and amazingly, they do this even in the summer! Some hapless people have even called my office to see whether I could advise them on the best number of treatments to take before vacations in order to "prepare" their skin for the onslaught of the sun while they're in the tropics! Needless to say, they got my 10-minute harangue on tanning, and a "Sun Cancer" handout sent right to their homes.

Interesting in this regard is that UVA, the supposedly "safe" wavelength of light that most of the booths use now, is *not* at all protective against damage from natural sunlight, or UVB. And we know that even UVB is damaging *enough*! So the theory that you can somehow protect yourself before a vacation by getting into the tanning booth is absolutely ludicrous. Remember that every photon of light that strikes your skin does a certain amount of irreparable damage—damage that will only appear as the wrinkles of your future.

No Safe Tans

A long time ago in my practice, a beautiful 16-year-old young lady named Leena came in asking for some routine skin advice. With her fair skin and blue eyes, I told her all the gentlest possible lotions and creams to use on her skin, along with a mild soap and, of course, one of the super sunscreens that I recommend routinely. During our discussion of her general skin care, I asked her about her plans for the upcoming summer vacation.

"Oh, I'm really looking forward to that, Dr. Bark. It's the first time I've ever had a summer job, and it ought to be tremendous fun!"

"What kind of job?"

"Well, my brother knows the manager of the city pool in our neighborhood." I began to hold my breath, almost knowing what would come next. "And I'm going to be a lifeguard! Isn't that wonderful?" I'm afraid she saw the openly chagrined look on my face right at that moment.

"I'm afraid it won't be the best thing to ever happen to *you* and your pale skin, Leena." I hardly knew what to say to her mother, who now was showing real concern as she listened. I decided to try to make good use of that concern, if I could. "You know what I'd do if Leena was my kid?" I asked her mother. "I'd *pay* her the same hourly rate she'd get at the pool just to sit home and read, rather than cook that gorgeous skin in the sunlight all summer!"

They both knew from the tone of my voice that I really meant what I was saying. That sun would predictably kill her lovely skin in a single summer, and for what? A little "tan," with which she wouldn't look all that good anyway, because of her normal light complexion? Hardly worth the wrinkles and skin cancers it would engender at a later date.

Happily, they listened to my advice and Leena worked in a library that summer. And when I saw that beautiful skin again in the fall, completely intact and lighter-toned than ever, I congratulated her on winning the struggle to save her face. If I could just get all the young women to listen so intently, I'd be perfectly happy.

The message here is that Leena's mom was interested enough in her to encourage her to listen to my advice.

And if she'd pay her *not* to work in the sun, I think many other parents ought to think about paying their kids *not* to get into the *sunbooths*!

So if you want to *guarantee* that your skin or your children's skin will really look old prematurely, try the tanning booths. But if you're interested enough to want to protect yourself against the onslaught of the sun, then avoid them with a passion. And join my "Tan Is Tacky" club, too. Take care of your skin—after all, it's got to last you a *lifetime*!

7

Retin-A and the Cancer Question

I've discussed the amazing abilities of Retin-A to cause "differentiation" in human cells. This means it makes cells that ordinarily would have become cancerous actually behave normally. It's been thought ever since the initial acne studies with Retin-A were done that that's why it works so well in acne. Acne patients have cells lining their oil gland openings that have not developed correctly—instead of flaking off and emptying out the oil gland openings as normal oil glands do, they stick together and form immovable clumps that plug up oil glands, making acne. Retin-A changes these *un*-differentiated cells back into normal cells that dump out of oil glands just as they are supposed to. Retin-A has properties that help acne, but this is the main one scientists think reverses the ravages of pimples.

But the work involving Retin-A and its relationship to cancer did not start with a study of acne. Researchers have known for years that lack of vitamin A, the basic parent compound of Retin-A, caused cancerlike growth in some animals. The reasoning went that if this were true, *adding* vitamin A, or chemicals that looked much the same but were less toxic to animals, would actually *reverse* cancer changes.

That would indeed work, but the problem was vitamin A toxicity—symptoms that would not be tolerated in humans, or would actually do harm to humans given high

═══════ *Youth Alert!* ═══════

Vitamin A–related compounds have been found, in experimental work, to prevent and even reverse some cancers. That is not a reason to begin taking extra vitamin A, because it is a toxic drug when taken in excess. Any extra vitamin A you take should be strictly under the advice of your personal physician!

doses of the compound. Those symptoms included redness of the skin and chapping of the lips, as well as extreme dryness of the lips, skin, and nose, and many others.[1]

Work progressed for many years involving virtually thousands of vitamin A–like compounds, and anti-cancer effects were discovered for many of these chemicals.

In the early years an initial fear of Retin-A developed: Doctors worried they might in fact be *causing* cancer in their patients by prescribing this drug for acne. Because Retin-A clearly does thin out the uppermost dead layer of the skin, dermatologists worried that sun damage would increase and therefore the patients on the drug would show higher numbers of cancers. The fact that some rats, overdosed on Retin-A, *did* get more tumors was hotly debated back in the early days of Retin-A therapy. In fact, the FDA put warnings on the package insert to state that such a finding had been noticed, and that patients should beware of exposing themselves to the sun while using Retin-A. This warning needlessly scared away many patients who would have benefited enormously from starting on Retin-A early in the course of their complexion problems.

That argument surfaced again as soon as Drs. Kligman and Vorhees discovered that Retin-A was useful in revers-

---

[1]Bollag, W. The development of retinoids in experimental and clinical oncology and dermatology. *Journal of the American Academy of Dermatology* 9:797–805, 1983.

ing the changes of radiaging. But the clear-cut evidence showed just the opposite changes took place while a patient is on Retin-A. *No* increase in cancers has *ever* been seen in patients on Retin-A for acne, and that's been quite a long time (about 20 years). If any problems were to have arisen from the use of Retin-A in humans, it certainly would have done so by now.

In fact, just the opposite is true: We see many *fewer* cases of skin cancer in people who have used Retin-A. In fact, studies are under way in several centers to obtain official FDA approval for a very special indication for the use of Retin-A: *reversal of minor premalignant changes in the skin!* Even more exciting news is developing about the "retinoids," the whole class of drugs based on the parent structure, vitamin A.

Many forms of cancer have been studied over the years to verify that Retin-A is an *anti*-cancer drug. Scientists have examined lung cancer in smokers on vitamin A, as well as bladder cancer and asbestos-related cancer, and have found vitamin A to lower the expected incidence of the disease.[2] Even breast cancer has been retarded by the family of retinoid compounds.

But even more exciting news is continually developing. Researchers are investigating the possibility that Retin-A may even *reverse* the preliminary changes of cervical cancer. Tests are ongoing now to prove that Retin-A, when applied in certain special ways by the patient to the uterine cervix, can normalize the Pap smears of women who would have otherwise required surgery.

Just what does all this mean? Will we all be on some nontoxic form of vitamin A in the future to ward off cancer? Are there, among the thousands of retinoid-like chemicals being tested, substances that will not harm us in any way, including the all-important side effect of fetal malformation? Could we even *hope* to see these developed

[2]P. M. Elias and M. L. Williams, Retinoids, cancer, and skin. *Archives of Dermatology* 117:160–75.

in our lifetimes? If the work concerning cervical cancer is any indication, I'd say we're all in for some astounding surprises in the field of retinoid therapy in the near future. The Retin-A you'll start as a result of reading this book is just the tip of the chemical iceberg. This may mark just the beginning of an age where chemistry won't be blamed for polluting people and their environment but rather will be credited with *saving* humanity from the ravages of cancer.

8

Can Retin-A Be *Your* Youth Miracle?

Retin-A's debut as the first real "cosmeceutical," a drug that *patients* could legitimately request for cosmetic reasons (versus the ones that the *doctor* prescribed on *his* initiative), was a turning point in the history of dermatology. Previously, patients came to the dermatologist asking for help for a problem—but they left the *type* of help up to him. Retin-A marked the first real departure from that age-old relationship, when people began to request a consultation primarily for the purpose of being put on a specific drug for aesthetic rather than medical reasons.

Some dermatologists, shocked by this departure from traditional medicine, and remembering stories of their internships and residencies when only a "druggie" or a neurotic would request a medicine *by name*, turned away from the drug and would not prescribe it for its anti-radiaging effect, even though they had used it for acne for many years! Clearly, both dermatologists and patients had a lot to learn about Retin-A.

I also think that this situation (of the *patient* requesting the drug) took some of the feeling of omnipotence away from some physicians, irritating them to the point that they disclaimed the drug, rather than be "forced" into prescribing it for the patients with radiaging who had courage enough to ask for it.

Youth Alert!

*Both physicians and patients are growing more and
more aware of how important appearance is to us all.
So don't be afraid to ask for Retin-A, and discuss it
freely and openly with your dermatologist.*

A Serious Prescription Drug

It should be eminently obvious at this point that Retin-A
is a serious prescription drug with many, many uses, even
though the FDA chooses to recognize it only for its effectiveness in acne. It should also be obvious that using it is
serious business, fraught with complications, which, while
easily handled in most patients, *do* in fact demand attention to the details of the treatment. It is *not* a "recreational" drug in any respect. Problems most often develop
if it is considered as such. Remember, drugs are put under
the aegis of the physician's prescription *because of serious
potential side effects*, and for no other reason. And while
the side effects of Retin-A are easily controlled if you have
professional advice, it *is* a powerful drug, and should be
treated as one.

Realizing that, you should also know by now that this
drug *does* exactly what dermatologic scientists say it does,
primarily, but not limited to, reversing premalignant skin
changes due to radiaging and effacing minor lines on the
skin surface. In the preceding chapters, I've explained a
lot of the science behind the Retin-A story just so you'll
be really prepared to use it intelligently, if you so desire.

Experience Is the Key

You also know how strongly I feel about proper dermatologic advice in the use of Retin-A. While the drug has

=== *Youth Alert!* ===

Please do not even try Retin-A if you're not willing to do all that's necessary to treat and protect your tender facial skin. Sunscreens and often moisturizers are essential, and sun avoidance mandatory!

been available and in active use by dermatologists for almost 20 years for the treatment of acne, most nondermatologist physicians actually have little experience with its use on a practical day-to-day basis—whether for acne or reversal of radiaging. And unfortunately, that includes plastic surgeons, who started prescribing this drug regularly only after the announcements in January 1988 that indicated Retin-A was effective in reversing minor wrinkles. What I'm saying here is that if you decide Retin-A is something you'd like to try, you should see the person who has dedicated his life to human skin and diseases of it, the dermatologist. To do otherwise is to cheat yourself out of the proper use of this medicine. It's truly a wonder drug, and understanding its effects, its complications, its dosage, its strengths and its weaknesses is the purview of the dermatologist, not your family physician, cardiologist, or obstetrician-gynecologist.

Your Drug, or Not?

So *is* Retin-A a drug for you, or not? Do you even need it? Do you want to put up with the minor hassles you've read about here, or would it be better for you at a later time? To answer these questions, you have to know a lot about yourself and your skin. Do you really have radiaging? When you look into the mirror in the morning, do you *really* see wrinkles, or just expression lines that are seen on all faces, depending on the way you are using your facial muscles

---

Youth Alert!

If you think about your wrinkles and/or aging once a day or more, you should seriously consider Retin-A.

---

at the time? Are you sun-damaged? We live, thankfully, in the "Sunscreen Generation," or what I *hope* will become so. Are you one of the leaders who found physical sun-screens (hats, long sleeves, other clothing worn in the sun) early on in life, and used chemical sunscreens (PABA and others) when they were developed? If so, it may not yet be your time for Retin-A. There really *are* people who *don't* need to use it—at least not yet in their lives—but it *is* legitimate for virtually anyone to start the medicine, if he realizes the side effects and cautions necessary for its use.

For what purposes do you want to use it? Are you look-ing for amelioration of your wrinkles, or for its anti-sun damage effects? Certainly it *is* legitimate to use this drug for wrinkles alone, since you still get the anti-cancer effects too, but there are many who need it for anti-cancer effect and *don't* use it just because they don't give a hoot about wrinkles. *They* really *should* be using it! That's where the experience of the dermatologist comes in. He will recog-nize that one simple fact and put those people on the drug who really *need* it, not only those who *want* it for reversal of wrinkling.

Are you willing to put up with the intense photosensi-tivity that Retin-A engenders? Can you really take my "Retin-A Pledge," and completely refrain from intentional sun exposure for the rest of your life (or at least for your Retin-A–using life, which should be one and the same)? This is the most serious challenge involved with using Retin-A. Do not remodel the front of your house (use Retin-A) while burning down the back porch (continue to get sun exposure).

Youth Alert!

Remember that Retin-A is not "kid's stuff." It is an important medicine and rejuvenator for your skin, and should not be taken lightly. I consider using it a lifetime commitment.

If you are *not* willing to take this important step in protecting your skin, you should tell your dermatologist that. There are other things you can do besides Retin-A, like acid peels, dermabrasion, collagen injections, and most of all, the use of sunscreens, which will at least *minimize* the damage of the sun, or repair some of the damage it has already done. Realize, though, that the surgical methods mentioned above are serious procedures that require some period of healing, and they are only one-time treatments—they do not keep working day after day to reverse aging effects in the skin, as Retin-A does. The message about sunlight and Retin-A is this: If you're not ready to swear off sun exposure, forget Retin-A!

Not Easy, But *Worth It!*

Are you willing to undergo some irritation for the ultimate help Retin-A can provide your skin? From reading about them here, you know some of the side effects you are apt to encounter with Retin-A. Will it upset you some mornings to go to work with a small amount of scaling on your face? What if you can't get your cosmetics on exactly as you'd like? Can you amend your old ways of cleansing and moisturizing to accommodate Retin-A treatment?

Are you willing to "push it" to get a result? In this regard, Dr. Vorhees, one of the pre-eminent Retin-A researchers, says that the more you use, and the more patiently you tolerate side effects, the greater and faster the improvement. Some of my patients tolerate this vigorous approach, and others—*many* others—do not. With them I must approach therapy with more time and most of all, more explanation and understanding.

An Answer, But No *Final* Answer

Is Retin-A the final answer? No, in several senses. No, in that there will be *other* retinoids, or vitamin A–like compounds, in the future that may be even better at reversing the cancerous changes of the sun's effect on the skin, as well as wrinkles. But those drugs are just in the preliminary phases of research, and it may be years before a practical substitute for Retin-A exists. And the point is this: If a patient comes to the doctor with strep throat, penicillin is the treatment of choice (in nonallergic patients). That's because there just doesn't need to be anything better! Penicillin works every time—there are *no* resistant strains of streptococcus, the bacterium that causes strep throat. That same principle holds for Retin-A: Although there can virtually always be *some* improvement on the currently available drugs, I'm not so sure we actually *need* another drug to substitute for Retin-A. It does what we want it to do, and it does it well. So don't count on 10 new drugs to take its place by the end of the decade—it just won't happen. This is the main argument for starting Retin-A *now* instead of waiting for something better to come along.

A rush of generic Retin-A's, however, is likely to come out within the next two years, because Johnson & Johnson's patent will shortly be running out. That usually means other companies will produce the same substance under different names. Whether they will be as good, or as reliable, or as stable as the original Retin-A will remain to be seen. I personally tried a variant of Retin-A produced by a West German company looking to get into the American market after the Johnson & Johnson patent runs out, but their form of Retin-A had an unusual odor and, I think, would be largely unacceptable to American patients who were accustomed to the fine quality and quality control of the Johnson & Johnson drug. In short, beware of substitutes for the real thing where Retin-A is concerned. You *may* be getting the real thing for less money—and then again, you may *not*. Are you willing to gamble with *your* skin?

Is Retin-A a cure-all? You already know the answer to that one. There is no free lunch, and no cure-all, either. Retin-A is clearly *not* the Fountain of Youth. No matter how hard you push it, and no matter how much peeling and irritation you tolerate, it will *not* correct the folds and deep creases on the skin. For that you'll need a team approach, involving your dermatologist and plastic surgeon. And in Part 2, you'll read about some of the other possibilities for improving your radiaged skin, and some special aging considerations.

Commonly Asked Questions

You may have heard the saying "There are no stupid questions—just stupid *answers!*" I'm a firm believer in that (in fact, I guess that's why I write books—to give some *straight* answers!). All patients, especially those embarking on a course of new drug treatment, should have *all* their questions answered, or else the doctor and his staff are not doing their jobs. As Dr. J. Graham Smith Jr. told me, "Joe, if your patient does something wrong, it's often your fault for not explaining it correctly."

Here are some commonly asked questions about the program and how it works. In the next chapter, we'll talk about the role of cosmetics in a program designed to reduce and reverse wrinkles.

Q: If I get all scaly and irritated using my Retin-A, should I just stop altogether? How should I handle this?

A: Scaling and irritation are a natural part of using Retin-A, so everyone should learn to expect these side effects to at least *some* degree, as we've already discussed in this chapter. No, you don't have to give up on the medicine—just stop for a few days, and when the scaling and inflammation go away, start again on a less frequent treatment schedule. For instance, when you *do* start to have excess redness, scaling, and tenderness, stop for two or three days, and then start back using the medicine, but at less frequent intervals. Often, it will be possible to restart the entire treatment program with just a little more adaptation time. In this way, I've been able to get most of the men and women who desire Retin-A to use it successfully.

Q: I have heard that Retin-A should be used differently in different parts of the country? True?

A: Some adjustments do need to be made in the Retin-A program, depending on where you live. One of the best summations of climatic conditions affecting Retin-A use was published in the November 1988 *Glamour* magazine. The article divided the country into six climatic zones, listing the problems associated with each zone, presenting "countermeasures" to keep the skin more normal while using Retin-A. Table 2 summarizes that excellent article, which drew on the sage advice of some of the nation's most respected dermatologists.

Q: I have a tanning booth in my basement that I like to use to stay brown all year. I've got fairly dark skin and have no problems with the sun, except for a few wrinkles around my eyes and mouth. Can't I go ahead and use my tanning booth, if I do it cautiously?

A: You just caused my heart to skip a beat! Do you know what you're saying? Chasing the "Great American Tan" while using Retin-A makes about as much sense as remodeling the front of your antebellum mansion while spraying burning napalm on the back porch! No problem with the sun? Sorry—your facial wrinkles are *proof* that sun has trampled over you and left its tracks. As I've said

Table 2   Climatic Effect on the Use of Retin-A

Type of climate	Problems	Solutions
Hot & humid	Skin may overheat. Sensitivity increases. Air conditioning dries skin more.	Don't overwash. Don't overuse cleansers. Use gentle soap or soapless cleansers. Use moisturizers and waterproof sunscreen. Excess oiliness may mean gel forms of Retin-A will be tolerated. Avoid applying Retin-A to skin folds—irritation may result.
Cold & dry	Lower humidity causes increased drying. Indoor heat is much drier.	Avoid *hot* water washes. Use a humidifier. Watch out for reflected and high-altitude sun damage.
High & dry	Altitude intensifies the sun's effect. Low humidity at high altitude increases dryness.	Use Cetaphil or SFC cleanser instead of soap. Use a moisturizing sunscreen (high potency) and a heavier, creamier moisturizer.
Cool & wet	Don't be fooled by clouds—UV rays penetrate well.	Use sunscreens; spot treat with moisturizers.
Temperate	Climate tempts you to stay in sun longer.	Use sunscreens with moisturizers.
Hot & dry	Increased irritation. Indoor air conditioning dries skin more.	Use very mild soaps. Avoid easily irritated areas like the nostril folds, upper lids.

many times, the only safe time to be in a tanning booth is at midnight with the plug pulled out of the wall.

Q: Really, now ... aren't they really *safer* than natural sunlight?

A: Hardly. We know that these booths emit high-intensity light and are more injurious than natural sunlight. Besides, we know they cause everything from drug eruptions in people on medicines for various medical conditions to skin laxity, ugly pigmentation, cataracts in the unprotected eye, herpes simplex and warts in people who lie upon those many-peopled, uncleaned surfaces, and now we even know that those radiation boxes cause big dips in the natural immunity to disease! Incredible to imagine how any thinking person could irradiate himself like that.

Q: But my husband and I have a boat and go to the lake frequently in the summer. Is it necessary to avoid what we consider to be the most fun of all, boating?

A: No, not at all. I'm a scuba diver as well as a dermatologist, and I'm often zipping out over sunny tropical waters, looking for another great dive site. Do you think I'm going to give up my diving fun? Not on your life. Over the years, I've instructed thousands of patients on "having their cake and eating it too." I dive and stay unwrinkled by using a waterproof sunscreen. As a matter of fact, as I write this I'm sitting by the sunny seashore (under a roof, naturally!) at a wonderful Caribbean resort. I stopped Retin-A about 10 days before coming here, and have been extremely careful on the dive boats to wear my highest-rated sunscreen and avoid all the sun that I can. *Still*, I had a slight sunburn on my forehead last night, after the first day of diving. And that's with a 29-rated sunscreen! So I *know* how sensitive to sun exposure Retin-A makes the skin.

Q: You haven't told me when I'll start seeing my wrinkles fade! Soon?

A: Well, don't look into the mirror each night expecting a magical result. Wrinkles fade, but not by any means overnight. It'll take 6–10 months to tell a difference in your wrinkles, even though most people say their skin feels tighter and firmer after just a few weeks of Retin-A. I *can* tell you this—after a year on the medicine, the little early wrinkles around my eyes (squint lines) are virtually *gone*.

Q: Can you stop applying Retin-A after the wrinkles fade?

A: We don't know yet. And the simple reason is that researchers have not been able to get anyone to *stop* the medicine! When a drug's effects are as impressive as those of Retin-A, and if the drug *is*, in fact, available by prescription for other uses, complete restriction of the medicine is almost impossible, without a group of extraordinarily cooperative test subjects. In short, some patients ask, "Do you think anyone in his right mind would stop this medicine?" It's a question that so far has only been answered in the negative.

The easier question to answer is whether or not the wrinkles corrected by Retin-A will return after the medicine is stopped. That would be a simple matter of biopsying a number of test subjects after stopping the medicine to see if the thickness of the dermis and the epidermis would return to its thinned-out, aged appearance. As I see it, two possibilities could occur. The collagen may thin back out with time, just as it did in the original skin under the influence of sunlight over many years, or it could remain the same thickness from then on if the person continued to avoid sun exposure. We have no idea yet as to which of these results we'll find, but one thing we do know for sure: The premalignant changes in the skin which would have, at some time in the future, formed frank skin cancers are now gone—wiped clean from the skin for a long period— probably, again, until enough damaging sun exposure (heaven forbid!) causes a whole new batch of lesions.

Q: Are there other uses for Retin-A, besides those you have discussed so far?

A: Absolutely! And now that you understand a lot more about the drug and its side effects, you should read Chapter 7 and the Appendix, concerning the other skin problems that can be effectively treated with Retin-A. Again, just as a reminder, none of these uses, except in acne, are approved by the FDA.

Q: I grew up with horrible cystic acne in the age before Accutane, the new anti-acne medicine. At that time, I resorted to whatever treatment my dermatologist could give me, including the meager antibiotics we had, and finally, on his advice, radiation therapy. Besides a thyroid cancer I've had removed years ago, I now have an incredible problem with my face, consisting of hundreds of scaly places that my current dermatologist calls "radiation spots."

My question is this: Is there any way to treat these spots (which the dermatologist says could turn to cancers with time) with Retin-A? Would it do me any good at all?

A: Absolutely! Retin-A could be the most important drug you've ever used, because of its wonderful properties of restoring order to the skin cells. It has the potential of reversing most of the skin damage done by the X-rays, if continued for a long time. Most of us would recommend that you start it gradually, as described in this chapter, and slowly increase the strength to the maximum tolerable, and continue that treatment for the rest of your life.

Of course, this is not guaranteed to remove all the spots forever. But it is an excellent place to start in chronic surveillance of your delicate radiaged skin. I can't tell you how crucial it is for you to watch this type of treated skin exceptionally closely. You truly have the potential for a disaster of major proportions: skin cancer or multiple skin cancers. Unfortunately, nobody knew that these problems would and could arise 20–40 years after the X-ray treatments. X-ray therapy for acne looked like a relatively safe way to save a teenager's social life. It's a sad story; it's result is that we must exert the maximum effort to watch for the constant possibility of skin cancers. To my mind, there'd be no better candidate for Retin-A.

Q: How about the cost of Retin-A? How long does a tube last? What about the Mexican stuff? Is the generic tretinoin they sell down there actually safe?

A: A tube of Retin-A cream, 0.05%, 20 grams, costs about $18–$20. Let's say it's $20. In the experience of my large patient series, a tube used on the face and tops of the hands lasts about two or three months. Thus a day's therapy costs about 22–33 cents. That's about a small pizza per month, and certainly a much better investment.

Is the Mexican tretinoin the same? Who knows? I cannot guarantee that the strength or chemical solution (one of the most important factors to consider in *any* topical skin treatment) would be anywhere near the same. My standard thought on generic drugs, and this would *certainly* apply to one possibly made by an unfamiliar foreign supplier, is that what's the use of paying less for possibly no effect at all? I don't think there's anyone who could seriously complain about the price of the medicine. So why waste the time with an unknown substitute for good-quality medicine? Still, there's always somebody around who'll try to beat the system.

Q: Should blacks think about using Retin-A?

A: The first thing to realize is that just as Caucasian skin isn't really white, black skin is not actually black. It is a mixture of various melanin types that result in a plethora of tonal variations to the skin.

My general advice would be to definitely consider using Retin-A if you are a very light-skin-toned black, or if you begin to show any of the conventional signs of aging, such as the fine wrinkles seen in Caucasian skin with increasing sun exposure. But definitely do use Retin-A if you work in an outdoor occupation and have had a lot of exposure to the sun. Even black skin with its superior sun protection can benefit from the healing and age-reversing benefits of Retin-A, if damage is occurring.

Q: Are there patients who just *can't* use Retin-A—whose faces, for some reason or another, are just too tender?

A: Not very many. Almost *every* person who really *wants* to try to adapt to Retin-A can successfully do so. But there are a few general categories of patients who probably should not be put on the medicine, or should be watched like a hawk if they *are* put on it. These categories include patients with the following diseases: lupus, rosacea, facial contact dermatitis (either irritant or allergic, at least until the eruption settles down), facial scleroderma, and a few other less common problems that make the face super-sensitive.

Part 2

Other Youth Miracles

9

Collagen and Other Filler Substances

Where does beauty begin and where does it end? Where it ends is where the artist begins.
—*John Gage*

Needless to say, Retin-A can't do it all. No one agent, technique, or operation can be expected to solve all the problems of aging, even if we *could* solve them all. But over the years some astounding developments have emerged from the laboratories of the basic scientists, who have made the day-to-day practice of dermatology and plastic surgery more exciting and rewarding. Among the basic discoveries that have helped us most is the discovery of substances called "filler substances," which can help us recontour the skin—to create smoothness where there was scar, beauty where there was deformity, and a youthful look where age had begun its inevitable assault.

Collagen: The First Approved Filler

In 1981, the first substance for the correction of inward defects in human skin was approved by the FDA for use by American physicians. It was an exciting time for all of us in dermatology. We badly needed some help with

=== *Youth Alert!* ===

Allergy to Zyderm Injectable Collagen occurs in only about 3% of patients. It's the most common complication, and prevents further use of the substance.

patients who had inward scars, defects, and wrinkles that required an implant to restore some of the thickness of the dermis.

The Nature of Collagen

Collagen is the leather of the skin. It's made in several forms by the body, and the amounts of the various types of collagen vary with the structure being studied. Collagen is basically a long-chain protein formed of three fibrils twisted in an elegant structure known as the triple helix. The fibers are made individually inside the cells of the skin known as fibroblasts, and upon secretion from the cells are hooked together at the ends, forming a sturdy, ropelike structure.

Long before the release of injectable collagen, it was discovered that human and bovine (cow) collagen are remarkably similar. The main differences lie in the end-pieces of the collagen fibers. It was this end-piece that long made bovine collagen unacceptable as an implant, because it regularly caused allergic reactions when injected into the skin. But chemists at the Collagen Corporation in Palo Alto, California, devised a way to clip off these allergenic ends of collagen molecules, making them suitable for injection into humans with an acceptably low incidence of allergy (about 3 out of each 100 patients are allergic to collagen). It was this advance that led to the release of the material for physician use.

Youth Alert!

The most common uses of Zyderm collagen in my practice are the correction of acne scars and the treatment of facial wrinkles.

Uses of Collagen: Many and Varied

Sometimes we think of collagen as being used only for aesthetic purposes in aging, such as injection of wrinkles to make them less visible in overhead lighting. But dermatologists have dreamed up many other legitimate uses, including the correction of acne scars, surgical scars that are depressed below the skin, and certain atrophies some people are born with. Some of these atrophies are very severe, involving fully one-half of the face, which is much smaller and sunken inward. Collagen has been a real lifesaver in these patients. It's also used to fill in the depression on the forehead produced in a strange disease called morphea. The lesion looks like the blow of a saber on the forehead, and thus is known as the "en coup de sabre" lesion. This deformity can also be nicely filled in with collagen.

But the lesion we're mostly concerned with in this book is the common age wrinkle in all its forms. It's the purpose of this chapter to tell you something about the appropriateness of collagen for correcting some of the types of wrinkles you may have. Then I want you to ask your dermatologist about the use of collagen and the other filler substances we mention here. Remember, not every dermatologist is skilled in the use of collagen injections, so you may have to search for someone in your area who does a good deal of collagen work to get a valid opinion about whether it will help in your case. Also remember that doctors sometimes tend to pooh-pooh those techniques about which they know the least, so you may have to do

> ═══════ *Youth Alert!* ═══════
>
> *Want the name of a dermatologist in your area who is skilled in collagen injection? Just call the Collagen Corporation's toll-free number, 800-227-8933.*

some looking before you find someone who knows enough to tell you all about it.

Types of Collagen

Collagen, under the brand names Zyderm and Zyplast, comes in several types, formulated for use in various areas of the face. Zyderm I, for instance, is injected into the skin as a test one month before the injections are done, just to make sure you have no pre-existing allergies to the substance. It is also used for the eye area wrinkles, but it is very thin and tends not to last very long in these areas, mainly because the type of skin there doesn't tend to hold onto the substance very well.

Zyderm II is thicker, and is used in superficial facial wrinkles to level them out with the skin surface.

Both Zyderm I and Zyderm II are un-cross-linked, which means the fibers are separate from each other, and when injected come into contact and link together into fibrils, the active agent in collagen injections. It's like a magic load of wood, which when thrown out onto the yard assembles itself into a house! But the fact that the fibers are individual and un-cross-linked means the body can reabsorb the substance fairly rapidly. We'll talk more about this later.

Zyplast, however, is partially cross-linked in the laboratory before it's injected. It's somewhat longer lasting and is generally used for the deeper areas of ridging and folding on the aging face, such as the glabellar crease

Youth Alert!

Zyplast is less likely to cause allergy than is Zyderm, because of its chemical structure.

(vertical line between the eyes) and the parentheses, or smile lines, arching around the mouth on either side.

It's an amazingly useful substance, which I use a great deal in my office. And we're finding other uses daily for this incredible form of implant, like re-establishing the "pout" on the upper and lower lip, in the areas called "Cupid's bow" in the center of the upper lip and the little bumps in the red area of the lower lip just on either side of the midline. You'd be surprised how many actresses have had this procedure done!

Zyplast can even be used effectively in the elderly for some annoying wrinkle problems. The best use in this age group is for "smokers' wrinkles," which run vertically and radially around and about the upper and sometimes the lower lips. It's possible to correct the main defects in the lip area using Zyplast, and Zyderm I or II to overlie the Zyplast and correct the superficial lines, for a fairly normal lip all your life, and that includes women smokers. Of course, collagen treatment in this area won't do the full job for those with ultra-deep wrinkles. In that case, plastic surgery may help restore the skin to near perfection.

Another common and very beneficial area to use Zyplast in the older population is in the "drooler's crease" along the corners of the mouth. This excess fold of skin where the lips converge is a common site for a minor yeast infection called perleche, which causes a chronic redness and soreness. A little Zyplast injected into those folds can open them up, flatten them out, and take away the nice moist hiding place for the yeast.

Safety Is Paramount

How safe is it to inject foreign protein into your body? Will it cause any other diseases in the future? What happens if you *are* allergic to collagen? All these questions are important for you to understand before you even consider collagen treatments.

With the most allergic ends cut off this molecule, collagen's threat of causing allergy drops dramatically. A few people *are* allergic to it, however, and show up with a positive skin test for the material when it is injected for the routine one-month test. When this happens, the injection site gets itchy and red, sometimes within 48–72 hours, but usually a positive test gets slowly redder over the first week or two after the injection. Dr. Arnold Klein, famed Beverly Hills cosmetic dermatologist and the largest user of collagen in the country, said at the 1988 national meeting of the American Academy of Dermatology that the best way to skin-test a patient to collagen is to do *two* skin tests in a row. In his method, the dermatologist does one skin test (always applied on the arm by the doctor himself to assure that it is put into exactly the right level of the skin), and reads it personally in three days. He then waits one whole month, and reads it again. If the test is still negative (as most are, of course), he applies *another* skin test, this time to the facial skin right up near the hairline, and waits two weeks to read the second one. If it's negative, then the collagen treatments are started. This is the best technique for testing collagen in your skin, and it's one I think you should insist on if you're going to get collagen treatments. This method assures the lowest possible number of reactions on the face when the treatments are begun.

Be aware, however, that even with a *negative* test, some few people, say 1 or 2 out of 100 in my experience, are still positive and produce a reddish reaction when the material is used on the facial skin. But most people are willing to risk this small chance of a red spot to finally have something that can correct some of their wrinkles.

There is no evidence that collagen causes other diseases or affects the body's immune system in any way. When a minor allergic reaction to the collagen in Zyderm occurs, it is a reaction to the cow collagen and not to the normal collagen present in the body. This means your body has formed antibodies against the cow collagen, but those antibodies will not attack your *own*, or "native," collagen. That's very important, because there are some diseases in humans called "collagen diseases," which we would want to make sure were not aggravated by the injection of collagen in its commercially available form, Zyderm and Zyplast. And keep in mind that if your doctor uses Zyplast, the thicker form of collagen, reactions are even *less* likely to occur.

Longevity of the Implants

Just how long do the collagen implants last? It seems that estimates of the longevity of the implants have shortened considerably over the years. When I started using collagen, we told patients it might last as long as 14–18 months, but we soon discovered that the material was reabsorbed faster than that. Current estimates for Zyderm I and II are about 6–12 months, but I commonly see good results longer than that, depending on the type of defect corrected and the amount of the material used.

Zyplast, in my experience, is a *somewhat* longer-lasting material. I'm convinced that it's present at least a year. This substance is truly a different product than the uncross-linked forms. Expect 6 months before touch-ups are needed, and then there won't be any surprises.

Amounts and Expense

The amount needed to fill in and smooth out wrinkles on the face varies widely with the type and size of the wrinkles present. There's no real way to estimate the amount you'll need on your own face. For this you must personally visit your dermatologist. And really, since prices for this material and the service of injecting it vary, quoting you prices for Zyderm and Zyplast would be difficult. I've personally seen them vary by as much as 150% in talking to my colleagues across the country.

What About Silicone?

Silicone is a very nonreactive substance derived from the second most abundant substance in nature, silicon, which is found in sand. It has been used for many years to make all types and sorts of medical implants. And true, pure liquid silicone is very useful for correcting minor skin defects such as acne scarring and wrinkles.

But the history of injectable silicone is studded with problems. Originally, an adulterated, contaminated form of the material was used, causing tremendous complications.

Currently, silicone is not approved for use in this country except by a very small group of investigators. The problem is that while this medicine is extremely effective in correcting minor skin defects, it has been overused. Too much silicone was used in a single procedure, or the time of waiting between treatments was not long enough. Problems also arose when materials were, in the past, added to pure, medical-grade silicone to "increase its effectiveness."

Needless to say, silicone really got a bum rap from all this, and indirectly, so did collagen. When "20/20" did a segment on silicone and its complications, they briefly mentioned collagen as a truly acceptable alternative, just before showing some really horrible pictures of complications from silicone. The next six to eight months saw requests for collagen drop to near zero, just because patients mistakenly associated it with silicone in that report.

The Future of Implants

Work is moving forward at a snail's pace to get the true medical-grade silicone approved for microinjection in the United States. It may come to pass, if the appointed investigators of silicone bring in a favorable final verdict. It would be extremely useful to have a material that could be used in cases of collagen allergy.

Currently, there's nothing else available except Fibrel, another form of collagen, which is mixed with the patient's own plasma for reinjection. And that particular substance is not warranted yet for use in wrinkles and lines on the face, but just for acne scars. Fibrel has an advantage over collagen, though: Its correction of defects in the skin is said to last a lot longer. Dr. Gary Monheit, chief researcher for Fibrel, says techniques are now being developed to inject this new medication more accurately into the wrinkle area, and it may soon be ready for use for this indication.

All the questions about implants are certainly not yet answered in this rapidly developing field. The only way you can get the correct opinion as to what's exactly right for *your* skin is to ask *your* dermatologist.

10

Plastic Surgeons: When to Go and How to Find One

Plastic surgery is not magic. No surgical procedure can restore lost youth or turn a fifty-year-old face into that of a twenty-year-old. Cosmetic surgery will not save a failing marriage or bring back a lost love, and changing a single feature will not transform you into a movie star . . . (but) it can give a lift to the inner self as well as the outer image.

—Paula A. Moynahan, MD, Cosmetic Surgery for Women

Plastic and cosmetic surgery is the fastest-growing medical specialty. In response to our quest for youth, the surgeons have nearly perfected operations that can lift our faces, suck our fat, straighten our noses, pin back our ears, make breasts bigger or smaller, revise our scars, tighten our lids, and a whole host of other important looks-related procedures for trying to attain some societal standard of beauty.

From personal experience, I can tell you the residency programs that train plastic surgeons simply cannot turn them out fast enough to keep up with the demand for their sophisticated techniques of body remolding. When a new one comes to town, it seems, even dermatologists have a difficult time getting our referral patients an appointment. But there are some really important general points you should know before you hop up on the plastic surgeon's table.

Before we get started talking about plastic surgery and plastic surgeons, let's talk a little about what this chapter *is not*. This is not a chapter all about the various options a plastic surgeon can offer you. For superb descriptions of plastics procedures and operations, their costs and complications, as well as exactly what you can finally expect from getting plastic surgery, I advise you to read the most important book on this topic ever written for the layman, Dr. Paula Moynahan's *Cosmetic Surgery for Women* (Crown, 1988), which is a national best-seller, and deservingly so. Written by one of only about 80 female board-certified plastic surgeons in this country, it is easily the best book about the subject ever conceived for patients. Incidentally, though the title suggests this is a book only for women, we know that more and more men are seeking plastic procedures all the time, and it serves them excellently as well. A copy of this book should be on the shelf of virtually *every* home library.

So rather than duplicate Dr. Moynahan's superb work (which I really could not do, nor would I try), I'll cover how I refer patients to plastic surgeons, in the hope that you'll at least be aware of some of the pitfalls of inexperience, credentialing, board certification, and the like.

When Should You Consider a Plastics Referral?

I'm often asked this question by patients with a rather embarrassed tone in their voices. And that always amazes me, that sense of guilt in asking about something to improve a patient's looks. It's as if our American work ethic makes us seem terribly vain if we show concern about our appearance and image. But I see this as a very *rational* concern—the concern for looking as good as we can for as long as we can.

```
=== Youth Alert! ===
```

If you look into the mirror closely one morning and notice your first sagging jowl, or deep crease, it's time to go see your plastic surgeon or your dermatologist for an evaluation. Acting in a timely manner will save you much pain in the long run. Keep in mind that going too early is much easier for doctors to deal with than "going too late."

So I'm very liberal and (some would think) somewhat forward in my recommendations about obtaining the advice of a skilled cosmetic surgeon. It's the same philosophy that applies to hair transplants and regrowth, leg vein injections, and all the other techniques this book discusses—the sooner the better. And this philosophy is what prompts me to tell a person next to me in the elevator that he has a skin lesion that needs to be checked. On the other hand, I'm very insistent that a patient not *push* for an operation *before* its time. You'll see this in a subsequent section of this chapter, "Six Rules for Finding the Right Plastic Surgeon."

What Is Plastic Surgery, Anyway?

Just for a second, put your fingers on the skin of your temple and move it around. See how far it moves, and how the skin around your eye is distorted when you do this? This is the skin's *plasticity* or movability, the chief characteristic that accounts for the term "plastic" surgeon, who is basically a surgeon skilled in the *movement* of skin and other tissues, like fat and muscle. I'm occasionally asked whether plastic surgeons use the substance *plastic* in their operations. Not at all, unless you interpret

Youth Alert!

"Plastic" surgery refers to the movement *of tissue, and the* minimizing *of scars.*

some of the materials they use to rebuild noses and other parts as "plastic" (they're really usually made of silicone, a nonreactive and safe substance that can stay in the skin for years).

Being skilled in the *movement* of skin, plastic surgeons can do what you could not do with your temple skin— move it without distorting another part of the skin. They have a host of incredible scientific methods of moving and reorienting skin to redrape it over the facial bones and other structures.

Is Plastic Surgery "Scarless" Surgery?

There's only one clear-cut answer to that question: *no*! A scar is made whenever the dermis of the skin is penetrated, and in surgery, that's every time. That simple fact should lead you to some important awareness of claims made by some surgeons. If a surgeon claims to be able to do surgery without scars, you should question him about this.

The principle of plastic surgery is to minimize and camouflage scars—to hide them inside hairlines and skin folds and natural wrinkles, so that they are *virtually* invisible. Yet if you looked closely enough, you could see even the most subtle of scars.

In short, scars are made every time the skin is penetrated.

===== *Youth Alert!* =====

In the final analysis, results are more important than credentials. But credentials are important as a starting point from which to evaluate a surgeon's expertise.

What About Credentials?

Before we talk about specific societies that endorse credentials of plastic and cosmetic surgeons, just how important is it that a surgeon is a member of one or the other certifying agencies? Isn't it all a big turf battle anyway, to see who gets the most operations?

Hardly. Most of these surgeons, in my experience, are so busy that they are looking for ways to *limit* their practices, and some take new patients only on referral from other doctors. Still, there is a sense of "turf battle" between the surgical subspecialists like ophthalmologists, ear, nose, and throat doctors (otorhinolaryngologists), plastic surgeons, and cosmetic surgeons. It would be far too easy to say that any doctor certified by the American Society of Plastic and Reconstructive Surgery is a "real" plastic surgeon and anyone certified by another agency is not, but that is far from the truth. Certainly, some minimal credentials should be held by each and every surgeon who attempts plastic and/or reconstructive surgery, but credentials are certainly not the whole story. We all know mechanics who claim to have been to all of a manufacturer's training schools on car repair who can't repair your car, but we also know a lot of people with uncertified mechanical skills who far surpass those others.

Ultimately, it's important to have an effective way to find a person you *trust* to do the job. And while nothing is foolproof except to the fool who believes it is, I use a

=== *Youth Alert!* ===

Want a great plastic surgeon? Ask your dermatologist
first!

few very effective steps that can lead you to a surgeon
who has skill and understanding.

Six Rules for Finding the Right Plastic Surgeon

1. *Ask your dermatologist* about the problem for which
you are seeking a consultation. Many times when this
happens I can tell a young woman that what she considers
to be a problem would do much better under the plastic
surgeon's knife in a few years instead of at this time. One
of the worst things you can do is seek an operation or
procedure before its time; the result is often that "oper-
ated on" look which tips everyone off to the fact that you've
had it done. Certainly this does not apply to things like
breast reductions and enlargements, otoplasties (ear repair
procedures), and others, but you've all seen the woman
who has gotten her eyelids done too early, or her acid peel
a few years before she would have needed it, and just looks
frankly unnatural. In my mind, that's much worse than
never having had the procedure in the first place.

The reason I say you should ask your dermatologist first
is that he's not standing there in the office with a knife in
one hand and a bill in the other, just as you enter the
examining room. Dermatologists see virtually *thousands*
of women who legitimately need plastic surgery, so we
know about the results that can be obtained and about
the look you can expect to achieve.

2. *Ask your friends* whether they have heard of the plastic or cosmetic surgeon your dermatologist has recommended. Don't be afraid to talk to them all about the procedure. You can save yourself a lot of wasted time in the doctor's office through the investment of a little talk over the back fence.

3. *Get a first opinion, get a second opinion, and get a third opinion.* Nothing could be more important. If you talk to several surgeons, you'll quickly get a feeling for the savvy of each, and whether or not you two are speaking the same language. It's impossible to overemphasize communication here. Remember that the person you're talking to will possibly hold a knife over your sleeping face, and if you can't trust him now, how can you trust him when it really counts?

4. *Try my "hands-off consultation" technique.* This is really worth the money you'll invest in it. Go to a surgeon and tell him that you're there to get his *opinion only*. Tell him you need to know the best ways to treat the problem or condition, but that he will *not* be the one doing the surgery. Now you might think this would be off-putting to a surgeon, but it's not at all. At least not to the best ones. Everyone appreciates a levelheaded, straightforward discussion of the need for surgery, and exactly what would be done in your specific case.

What's the effect of this? Freed from any financial expectations, the surgeon you see under the "hands-off consultation" rule will often give you a wonderful idea of all the possible techniques that could be used to correct the problem. You'll get all his literature about the procedure you need, which may, in itself, tell you something about his concern for patients and his professionalism. Some of my happiest patients were those who did just this. Then really do keep your promise to yourself to see the two other surgeons, *no matter how fantastic the first one sounds*. I've had patients say they've seen striking differences in techniques when they did this, and some have

---

Youth Alert!

Nobody's got a lock on an ethical *technique. Remember that. And if anyone tells you he's the only one who does a certain procedure, ask some more questions. Any medical procedure is available to all doctors and surgeons, not just the one who tells you about it first.*

---

delayed their surgeries for extended periods in order to find a surgeon with whom they are compatible.

A final word about the "hands-off approach" to finding a great surgeon. If you talk to two or three surgeons, and you seem to like the first person best, you can still go to him for the surgery, even though you told him he would not be the one doing the operation. Again, honesty is the best course here—just explain to him that after checking out several others, he seemed the best and most compatible with you and your required operation or procedure.

5. *Make sure you see actual "before and after" photographs* of each surgeon's own patients, and ask how many of this type of operation he's done. Ask for names of 5 or 10 patients you could talk to about how things went. You really *can* do this! I maintain a file of patients in my office whom I can call on to explain a procedure to a potential patient who needs it. The one that comes to mind immediately is circumcision in an adult male. This needs to be done sometimes because of occasional infections that can occur, but patients dread the operation so much that I've found it helpful to have them talk with someone who has had it done. I have such a patient who has agreed to help me out with this from time to time, and prospective patients are very glad to discuss it with someone who has had the operation. You can do the same thing with the plastic surgeon's patients. If he won't introduce you to some folks who will talk about the procedure, keep looking for a doctor who will.

Youth Alert!

Ask to talk *to some patients who have had your intended procedure. To rely only on photographs can be very risky!*

My office has this same kind of file of patients who have had all the various plastics operations too, and who have agreed to talk to someone considering the same procedure. But it's much wiser to get names of people directly from your plastic surgeon—the one who will finally do the surgery.

The other part of this tip is more delicate. You should see some photographs of complications too. To see only the good results is unrealistic, and most surgeons will be amenable to showing you some of the minor and major complications that can, in a rare case, happen. We do this routinely in our office with leg vein injection therapy (sclerotherapy), for which we have an extensive collection of my own patient slides and those of world-renowned expert Dr. David Duffy. Keep in mind that you should always be made fully aware of what you're getting into.

6. *Don't you dare be rushed into anything.* It's vital with all surgery, except critical emergency operations, that you and your spouse or friends have a chance to talk it over in the calm, unpressured atmosphere of your own home. *Never* have a cosmetic procedure done the day you go in for the consultation. Things can look a whole lot different later, and you may live to remember with chagrin the old saw, "act in haste and repent at leisure!"

I realize that this discussion of all the effort you must go through can scare off some patients who really could benefit from cosmetic surgery, but I feel it's necessary to consider these things before the fact.

If plastic surgery sounds scary, it shouldn't. It should, however, sound *serious*, and should never be approached

---

====== *Youth Alert!* ======

If you rush into a plastic surgical operation without discussing it with your "significant others" and your dermatologist, you may create more problems than you'll solve.

---

lightly. If you do this with your eyes fully open, and with adequate preparation, as you would receive from Dr. Paula Moynahan's book (*Cosmetic Surgery for Women*), you can have a successful procedure with the greatest chance of no surprises. That's what's most important, and that's why you should take all these precautions.

11

Liposuction: Getting the Fat Out of Your "Pockets"!

Beauty is a greater recommendation than any letter of introduction.
—Aristotle

Any book dealing with youth and ways to retrieve and maintain it would be incomplete without mention of fat suction surgery, one of the most popular operations in history. It has nearly surpassed 100,000 cases in just the United States in 1988, topping breast enlargement in total numbers for the first time. I was determined, since I am neither a cosmetic surgeon nor a surgically oriented dermatologist, not to comment extensively on the actual technical aspects of the operations that are performed by those physicians. This has been done in wonderful thoroughness elsewhere, such as Dr. Paula Moynahan's *Cosmetic Surgery for Women*.

But the science of dermatology so closely interweaves with plastic surgery, and fat suction surgery is so immensely popular, useful, and successful, that I felt it necessary to comment on its appropriateness in several major aspects.

First of all, you should realize that liposuction surgery (otherwise known as lipolysis) is a relatively new procedure. For instance, in the United States it has only been used for about six years. And although it has been used

================ *Youth Alert!* ================

Realize that liposuction, although performed often in this country, is a fairly new procedure. Some areas of liposuction on the face, for instance, are considered investigational.

in Europe for quite a bit longer, as a valid surgical procedure it is still in its infancy. That, to me, is reason for due *caution*—not reason enough not to *have* this type of procedure done, if you need it, want it, and realize what you're getting into.

Some Details of the Procedure

Liposuction is performed with a steel cannula (hollow tube with a hole at the tip), which varies in size, depending on the area to be treated. Larger areas with coarser fat are treated with a larger-diameter cannula, and smaller areas, like the area under the chin, are treated with a very small tube. It's this advance of smaller cannulae that has led to the beautiful results we see these days from liposuction surgeons.

The tube, which is connected to a machine that can produce powerful suction, is inserted into a small incision made in various parts of the body that have pockets of excess fat. These can include the chin, thighs, abdomen, "saddle bag" areas of the hips, "love handles" on the waists of men, knees, and even the *ankles*! Almost any area that has excess fat is a logical candidate for liposuction. The incisions themselves are extremely small, and thus spare the patient long, spread scars common with other types of fat removal procedures. The aim of liposuctionists is to make only those scars that would be difficult to find if you were examined in the nude.

Youth Alert!

You are not going to lose weight *by having a liposuction procedure—only isolated, unsightly pockets of fat.*

Almost all patients are treated as outpatients, having the procedure and going right home afterward. The patient is often given a general anesthetic, because there can be significant pain involved with the suction of the fat. Fat is withdrawn in a "honeycomb" pattern, which produces multiple small tunnels that slowly collapse as the fat is withdrawn. This collapse of the honeycombed areas is what causes the flatter, less bulging look of areas treated with liposuction. Bleeding and fluid loss are usually minimal, and patients generally recover very quickly and completely from the surgery.

Often special compression garments (some look like very heavy girdles) are advised for a matter of weeks or months, in order to get the tissues that have been disrupted to knit back together. This is very important to avoid "bagging" of the skin after liposuction.

Not a Weight-Control Technique

Although liposuction has many positive aspects, in terms of the obvious improvements in appearance from eliminating pockets of fat, you should realize that one of the things it *can't* do is function as a weight-loss regimen. No one would approach liposuction as a method of weight control, because surgeons cannot remove *that* much fat. This procedure is for *localized* pockets of fat. It is *not* a substitute for diet and exercise. The maximum that can be removed at any one time (by conservative surgeons) is about 2,000 cubic centimeters (about 2 quarts of fat).

Timing Liposuction

And while on the subject of weight loss, we should consider the question of when it is appropriate to have liposuction surgery. Should a person, for instance, be required to get down to his optimum weight before having the operation? Since many could never reach and hold their optimum weight, this is probably not a legitimate requirement. It is more logical to require a person to attain the lowest weight he can reasonably expect to maintain, and then go ahead with the operation. But most of the people who have liposuction are not the grossly obese. In fact, noted plastic surgeon Dr. Martin Luftman of Lexington, Kentucky, considers obesity a *contraindication* to liposuction. He uses it mostly in people with what he calls "disproportionate fat." That is, a normally well-contoured individual would have liposuction to remove isolated areas of ugly fat that can't be lost through diet and exercise.

As Dr. Luftman says, "It's not possible to hook someone up to a suction machine and drain his whole body!" But it is possible, says Dr. Luftman, to stage the procedure so that much more fat can be removed at later times. This is what makes it possible to do the "saddle bags" on the thighs, for instance, or the buttocks, which often require more than one procedure. Surgeons are wise to plan more than one procedure for difficult cases of liposuction. Such staged procedures generally result in a smoother overall correction of the fatty area. Dr. Luftman estimates that fully a third of patients undergo more than one procedure. "It's better to touch up the treated area with a minimal procedure later than to take out too much on the first surgery," he says.

Liposuction is no minor surgical technique. It is said to be limited only by the safe volume of fat that can be removed, and by the strength of the surgeon, who has to push and pull the cannula through the body. That second limitation, physical endurance of the surgeon, is com-

---

Youth Alert!

One medicine that a liposuction patient must not have within at least 48 hours of the operation is aspirin. *This, plus other anti-coagulants, can intensify bleeding at the time of liposuction surgery.*

---

monly mentioned in many of the references to liposuction surgery in the medical literature, which should indicate that all in all, it's pretty tough on the patients too, when larger areas like hips, buttocks, and thighs are done.

Complications

While the photographs you may see of liposuction results may, in and of themselves, be dramatic, that does *not* mean *everyone* achieves such results. And the larger the pocket of fat, the more chances for complications. Some of the many complications that have been reported with liposuction surgery include the following: bleeding; numbness of the skin in the fat-sucked areas due to disruption of the nerves leading to the skin in the fatty areas; sagging of the skin postoperatively in patients who had inadequate skin tone to begin with or who did not follow the advice of their surgeons to wear the compression garments for the right length of time; actual necrosis or loss of patches of skin in the areas; embolisms (injury to the lungs or other body part, due to the traveling of bits of fat through the bloodstream), and death. But I want to make it perfectly clear that this is one of the safest operations a person can have, and these complications are extremely infrequent. In short, in the right hands, liposuction can be a real godsend.

Finding a Surgeon

The first thing to do when you're looking for a good plastic surgeon for liposuction is to read Chapter 10, "Plastic Surgeons: When to Go and How to Find One." And consider careful questioning of the surgeon, using the techniques I outline there. Think of this. Liposuction has only been used for about six years in this country, and while all the plastic surgical residencies now train their candidates in this technique in detail, most of the plastic surgeons who now *do* this procedure were *not* trained in it in their residencies! How, then, did they learn it? By extensive postgraduate courses in the technique, and by attending patients in the offices and clinics of more experienced surgeons who have done many of the procedures. It *is* legitimate, however, to *ask* your prospective surgeon just how much training he has had in the technique. Again, many of these points are outlined in Chapter 10.

Approach liposuction as you would any other procedure done on your body: with your eyes open, and your questions ready!

12

It's Not Vain to Hate Your Veins

Please, Dr. Bark, can't you do something about my "purple malaise"?
—A leg vein patient

It's an all-too-common story. A woman, reaching thirty-something, goes on vacation, then bursts into my office on her return.

"Dr. Bark, I just can't believe how bad my legs look!" exclaimed Marla, a longtime friend and patient. "We went down to the beach for our yearly outing with the kids, and when I put on my bathing suit, I was too ashamed to go out with my legs showing!"

"Ah yes," I said, examining the reddish-purple spider veins in her legs. It looked as if a young child had gone berserk on her skin with a purple felt-tipped marker. "I can understand your feelings about not wanting to wear a suit. How long have they been like this?"

I knew that Marla had three strapping young boys, and that she had been taking birth control pills after the birth of her most recent one. She was approaching 40, and I had advised her some time ago, for an acnelike eruption, to consider stopping the pill for just such reasons. She had not.

====== *Youth Alert!* ======

The most common causes of expanded, ugly leg veins are genetics (inheritance), hormone adminis- tration (for example, the pill), trauma to the legs, and the normal amount of circulating estrogen women ordinarily have.

"They've been there for years to a minor degree, but recently they've really exploded. They're broken veins, aren't they?"

Common Causes of Unsightly Veins

I went on to explain to Marla that the veins she could see so prominently in her legs were not really broken. The blood was still flowing in them, and that's why they looked so ugly and prominent. In fact, they were caused by years of exposure to the hormones involved in just being a woman, and were not helped at all by bearing children and taking the pill, both of which increase estrogen levels.

Estrogen, the female hormone, is well recognized to cause a general growth of small blood vessels. That's why we see far more of these so-called spider veins on the faces and legs of women than we do in men (but more about this later in this chapter). I'd estimate the ratio at about 50:1, women to men, indicating the strong hormonal link.

The lesions on the face are most commonly treated in the dermatologist's office with a special form of electric needle, which seals them for good in just a few short treatments. It's the legs that are the real and lasting scourge for women who are trying not to look their age. Actually, I decided to include this chapter because so many women tell me that they can't *feel* young, no matter how many fine lines on their faces are eliminated by Retin-A and other means, if their legs still look so bad. Most of you who either have such veins or have seen them on the legs of your mothers, sisters, friends, or relatives will understand.

My examination of Marla showed about a dozen dark bluish-purple superficial areas of veins that stood out horribly on her legs. She was disgusted by them, and clearly would have done almost anything to get rid of them. She had even invested in coverup-type leg cosmetics for months, but finally gave up on this tack, because they are so miserably hard to put on the wide areas of leg skin that must be treated. So most women turn to longer dresses and slacks to hide their blemished legs.

Let's look at the main types of veins and what we can do to help them.

Leg Veins and Treatments

Although the experts classify veins in the legs in many ways (according to size, color, anatomical structure, and location), for purposes of discussion here, we'll talk about the two main types on the legs that cause problems. The first type are the ones Marla has, the dark red to purple "starburst" veins that are often visible from virtually *yards* away. Old-time physicians used to tell women that these were caused only by pregnancy, resulting from the slowing of blood return from the legs because of the downward pressure exerted by the fetus on the veins in the abdomen. For years this seemed a plausible explanation, until the relationship between estrogen and blood vessel growth was firmly established.

But what can be done for them? A technique called sclerotherapy has been developed, in which these dilated, useless veins are injected with various solutions that cause them to be reabsorbed. This happens because the injected solution irritates and begins breaking down the wall of the vein. Blood flow stops as a thrombus, or tiny clot, forms inside it. The vein is then turned into a "cord" of

---

Youth Alert!

Ask *your sclerotherapist what solution he's using for your veins. If he says sotradechol, beware of the complications of this medicine.*

---

blood and fibrous tissue that slowly gets reabsorbed by the body, leaving an area of normal-looking skin.

Sclerotherapy solutions have been developed that are supersafe and which will result in complete obliteration of the visible veins on the legs. But you should know that some of the solutions are safer than others.

The principle solutions are *sotradechol, hypertonic saline,* and *aethoxysclerol.* Probably the most commonly used solution is sotradechol, a powerful vein-treating substance, most often used by vascular surgeons and other nondermatologists. It is FDA-approved, but I do *not* advise its use. Deaths have occurred with this solution, even though it happens to be the only FDA-approved substance for sclerotherapy. The bottom line is this: I'll be glad to let you use something that will correct the vein problem, but I'll not advise you to be injected with a potentially lethal product, FDA-approved or not!

That leaves two solutions in common use by dermatologists, many of whom are members of the North American Society of Phlebology (a society of professionals who perform sclerotherapy of veins—more about this society later). The more commonly used of these two remaining solutions is hypertonic saline (strong salt solution), which, in the right hands, is very safe for vein injections. Established, experienced practitioners of sclerotherapy favor it, for several reasons. One is that no allergies to this medicine have been reported. That alleviates a lot of fear on the parts of the doctor and the patient undergoing the injections. And let's face it, many patients do have multiple allergies to medicines of all types these days, and it's

Youth Alert!

Beware that complications exist for any technique, even when the safest solutions are used. It is up to the physician to make you aware of the complications, but it's your skin, so make sure you ask about them and that you understand all the known risks involved. This cannot be overemphasized.

very nice to know that one solution exists for leg vein injections which is safe, even in those allergic patients.

Hypertonic saline is available in the United States, even though it has no approved indication for vein removal. It can cause stinging on injection and very frequently causes leg cramps, probably because of the minor changes occurring in the leg muscles from the small amount of salt injected. It also requires strict precision on the part of the physician/injector, because if any of this solution gets out of the vein into the surrounding skin, a small ulcer often results. If the dermatologist notices that a small amount has gotten outside the vein into the skin, he will inject the area with normal saline (a weaker salt solution that the body tolerates perfectly) to dilute the stronger salt solution, thereby frequently preventing the ulceration. Still, you must realize that this can happen, and if an ulcer *does* develop, a small ivory white scar may be left in the area permanently. (However, in the cases of scarring after a minor ulceration that I have seen, the final result is *much* preferable to most women than was the original vein— still, it's an occurrence we always try to avoid.)

The other solution in common use is aethoxysclerol (EOS), which is not FDA-approved but has been used safely by experts for many years. It may be the safest solution of all, and it's the one that's always advised in training new dermatologists to perform sclerotherapy. That's because ulcerations and scarring almost never occur with EOS, which means a minor injection of some of the solution outside the target vein is of no consequence. Also, it's much less painful, because the medicine, which is imported from Germany, France, and England, was originally designed as an anesthetic. But when its tests as a local anesthetic began, it was found to irritate and seal blood vessels, so it was abandoned for that use and adopted for use in sclerotherapy, where it works like a charm.

You're probably wondering whatever became of Marla's veins. I treated her set of about 12 small starburst veins in three sittings, covering what sclerotherapists call one "session" per sitting, consisting of about 12 minutes a session. She was treated a total of three times for each target vein, over about a three-month period, and had about an 80% improvement. Now it was possible for Marla to walk on the beach again without fear that everyone was staring at her legs, except that they really are attractively shaped, and now she's proud to show them off!

Treating Varicose Veins

But what about the larger veins on the legs, the ones for which *color* is not so much a problem as the fact that they protrude from the skin, sometimes quite prominently? These are the veins that we commonly refer to as *varicose*. Amazingly, even these larger and deeper veins can be treated with injection therapy, but with a slightly more difficult technique and with special precautions after the injections, like pressure bandages taped over cotton balls in the areas of the injections, and even sturdy support hosiery to help the legs recover without subsequent irritation and soreness.

The injections, even with large vessels, result in rapid reabsorption of the veins themselves. For these larger, thicker veins, a larger quantity of the solution is injected, and complete reabsorption of the destroyed vein takes a lot longer, mainly because we're talking about a much larger physical mass of tissue your body must reabsorb.

Youth Alert!

Large and small veins can be obliterated by injection therapy. Always investigate this safe alternative to surgery before consulting a surgeon.

In other words, don't expect sudden miracles. Expect that follow-up treatments will be necessary.

Tips on the Treatments

How should a woman prepare for the vein injection session? I'll give you a few of the tips I learned from the master in the field, Dr. David Duffy of Torrance, California, who taught me the art of sclerotherapy. As with any medical procedure you have planned, however, you should always call the office of the doctor you've selected to treat your veins and ask for any special instructions concerning the treatments. Often, as in Dr. Duffy's case, you'll be advised to do certain things, like:

Wear shorts. For obvious reasons, it makes treatment much easier, since frequent turning and repositioning is necessary on the treatment table.

Don't apply any lotions the day of your appointment. Doing so causes your legs to be too slippery, even when the dermatologist cleanses them with alcohol. It's often necessary for him or his assistant to stretch the skin firmly, in order to pin down the tiny vessels he'll be injecting, so be patient with all this.

Don't use a creamy "beauty bar" for washing on the morning of the treatment. Again, to do so can risk slipperiness on the leg skin, due to the oils put into such bars to moisturize the skin. Ordinarily, I would *advise* such soaps, but not on the day you receive your leg vein injections.

══════════ *Youth Alert!* ══════════

It's extremely important for you to follow your own doctor's list of instructions about care of your legs before and after undergoing sclerotherapy. His word is law in that regard. The suggestions made here are only to help you understand the process and to visualize it.

Eat something prior to having your legs injected. All doctors know that some of the biggest football players we've ever treated have keeled right over in our office hallways after getting a very small shot of some medication. The principle's the same for you: You *must* eat, especially if you're going to have a procedure done or blood drawn. I've been constantly amazed at how well this helps patients avoid fainting.

Continue to exercise after the injections are done. This will help prevent the minor superficial thrombophlebitis, a soreness in the skin where the veins have been injected. It is often recommended that patients walk a mile each day for a couple of weeks after the veins are injected, and I personally advise my patients to do exactly that. Make sure you ask your own doctor for his instructions about exercise, and follow his program exactly!

Do not shave your legs on the mornings of your treatments. You may consider yourself a competent and careful shaver, but every shave results in small cuts on the skin, which burn like fire when the dermatologist spreads layer after layer of alcohol on the legs to best visualize the tiny veins. If you shave, you'll regret it, and it may, in fact, make it too painful to complete the procedure.

Fees and Insurance Reimbursement

How much does all this cost, and how do you go about finding a dermatologist who uses the right technique and the best and safest solutions for obliterating your veins? Cost is the hardest consideration to discuss, because professional fees vary so much across the country. Generally, however, I'd estimate somewhere between $100 and $200 a session, keeping in mind that a "session" is about 12 to 20 minutes long in most offices, and during this time the doctor will do as many veins as he can safely treat. I realize that is quite a spread between the high and the low figures; the only way you can be sure of the costs is to call the dermatologist you plan to use and ask him for an exact quote for the charges.

Most physicians who do this procedure do have an appropriate insurance code for sclerotherapy for "painful leg veins." Pain is a legitimate reason to treat leg veins and a frequent finding in the types of varicosities (abnormally enlarged veins) for which you would seek sclerotherapy. That means a significant number of, but certainly not *all*, patients receive insurance reimbursement for treatment of their veins. That's good news for your legs *and* your pocketbook! You should ask your dermatologist carefully about his ability to obtain insurance reimbursement for his sclerotherapy patients in the past, and that will, of necessity, color your decision of choice of doctors to do the job. Realize, however, that the prime consideration in treating your veins is the *final result*: Obliterating your veins safely and effectively should be paramount, and price considerations secondary.

Facial Veins and Their Treatment

We've discussed the veins in the legs and their treatment, but what about those in other locations? I've seen experts in this procedure inject veins that were actually *tinier than the needle with which the injections are done*! And while this is the exception rather than the rule, many, many types of venous lesions on the skin can be done with this technique. The most common places it is used are in the

nonfacial areas. The facial areas are less apt to respond
to the *injection*-type therapy, and more likely to do best
with what dermatologists call electrodesiccation (ED
treatments).

Expanded blood vessels on the facial skin can occur in
both women *and* men. In women, they are largely attributable to radiaging and estrogen exposure over years and
years, but in men (and occasionally in women too) they
tend to be caused by heavy drinking (and smoking), and
they are also seen in those with a fairly common skin
disease, rosacea, which makes the capillaries on the face
enlarge greatly.

Treatment of rosacea usually consists of oral tetracycline and topical sulfur and hydrocortisone preparations,
as well as avoidance of certain chemical and physical factors, such as weathering (sun, wind, heat, cold), caffeine,
drinking hot liquids (perhaps the greatest stimulus to its
formation), and possibly eating spicy foods, although some
investigators deny this is a factor. Note that on rare occasions, enlarged facial vessels can also result from certain
important internal diseases, like lupus erythematosus, liver
diseases, and others. Your dermatologist will talk to you
about these conditions, and possibly test for them, too.

But more often than not, treatment of rosacea will not
result in the complete resolution of the enlarged facial
blood vessels. That's where ED enters the picture, even
for men—men who want to maintain their youthful
appearance, that is.

Youth Alert!

Rosacea is a vicious, chronic disease, consisting of bumps and pustules in the central face, accompanied by redness of the skin and blood vessel overgrowth. It's a highly treatable condition, and now we can even remove the expanded blood vessels which are the hallmark of this condition.

Electrodesiccation

ED treatment is a simple form of cautery done with an extremely fine platinum needle that is carefully directed with appropriate magnification through the epidermis right down onto the vessel. Then, when a small electrical current is applied, the vessel is sealed shut, or cauterized, by the heat produced. The technique stings a tiny bit, but not enough to require any anesthesia—in fact, injecting numbing medicine into the areas to be treated with ED will often make the vessels disappear, rendering the treatment useless.

Results? In skilled hands (and *most* dermatologists are experts at this procedure for facial blood vessels and "broken" capillaries), these annoying reddish spots can be removed beautifully while leaving almost no sign that an ED procedure was ever done. Sometimes, however, ED can leave very tiny dots in the area where the needle burned not only the vessel but a minuscule amount of the delicate facial skin overlying it. This is sometimes an indication that a slightly higher current setting was used than would have been necessary.

You should have a few test spots done first, before doing a faceful of vessels (a great idea for any widespread procedures or procedures in cosmetically important areas, so that you can test the doctor and he can test your skin!). In this way, you should be able to show him any tiny marks left so that he can decrease the current in the elec-

=== *Youth Alert!* ===

*If you have any doubt about how your skin will toler-
ate any new procedure, ask that a small, inconspic-
uous test area be treated first. Then you and your
doctor will be better able to evaluate the technique
with your particular skin. Remember, all treatments
are not alike for all skin, skin type, or patient.*

tric needle the next time and make spots that are nearly
invisible.

The prime indication for which I perform the ED procedure is the tiny capillary spiders on the facial areas and
neck, most often near the nose and cheeks, where radiaging, genetics, estrogen, rosacea, other diseases, and time
tend to enlarge these vessels. Sometimes they get so large,
they can make the entire face look red! In these cases, the
ED procedure makes life livable again.

But ED is not suitable for all areas. On the legs it's not
at all suitable, because of the dots and scars left after the
sites heal. These marks, often permanent, can be seen
every few millimeters or so along the course of the blood
vessels where the procedure was done. For the legs, sclerotherapy is *vastly* superior! Don't let *anyone* use ED on
your leg veins.

=== *Youth Alert!* ===

*Be aware that there are a few serious medical dis-
eases that can cause these vascular spiders and
enlarged blood vessels to appear on the face. Your
doctor will question you about these, and possibly
obtain tests to exclude these illnesses, if he deems it
necessary.*

Youth Alert!

Beware of the "fool with a tool," a doctor who claims to be able to do almost every procedure with his "pet" technique (laser, or whatever!). Each technique generally has a few very limited applications, and you should ask other specialists for a second opinion if you suspect you are being sold a bill of goods about the use of any one method.

The "Fool with a Tool" Problem

Talking about techniques brings to mind the "fool with a tool" risk. It is very important for you to avoid seeing any doctor who claims to be able to remove facial and leg veins with a laser. Especially beware of those you see actually *advertising* such procedures, or someone who claims to perform all such procedures with a laser or any other single modality to the exclusion of all other techniques. Lasers have very limited application; and those include such lesions as port wine birthmarks and some facial vascular spider-type lesions (especially when an entire *area*, like the whole nose, is involved). It is not, generally, a tool with which to remove cancers or moles, because of the destruction of valuable tissue needed for pathologic study, and certainly not for removal of leg veins, where ugly streaks of pigment and even scars can result from the intense heat of the laser light.

Some practitioners have purchased lasers and feel they have to use them for more indications than are warranted, because the expense of the machine is so high, more procedures are necessary to make the machine pay for itself. I'm not accusing all laser surgeons of such dubious ethics, but indeed there are a few bad apples in every barrel who can spoil a wonderful tool for selected applications for all of us.

It's like the silicone controversy (see Chapter 9): The material was used inappropriately in many cases, which killed its chances for being used anytime in the future for indications that were proper. Just be careful. Such caution will protect you from unethical practitioners, and protect good and warranted treatments from getting an undeserved bad reputation that could prevent their use in conditions for which they *are* warranted.

Where can you get further information about leg and facial vein treatments? First, ask your dermatologist. He'll either do it himself or send you to someone locally who can do the injections correctly, and with the best technique and solutions. In any specific area, there are often doctors who are well-known to the medical and dermatologic community who do the sclerotherapy procedure. If talking to your own dermatologist about it doesn't help, you can try our national organization. Just write the North American Society of Phlebology for recommendations on a specialist in your area. The address is:

> North American Society of Phlebology
> P.O. Box 1054
> San Diego, CA 92075
> 619-942-0924

Commonly-Asked Questions About Leg Vein Treatments

Q: How many sclerotherapy treatments are necessary to clear up my awful-looking leg veins?

A: We usually estimate that three to five treatments will be necessary, most often on one of two schedules. The more common schedule is injection of the veins in all accessible areas about every two to three weeks, for as many as five sessions. Many of the vein-bearing areas will be injected multiple times, and even if they are not completely invisible at the end of the fifth session, they do usually keep fading out to invisibility.

Often, after three to five sessions, we give a patient a rest period of 3 months or so and then reinspect the veins. This gives them a chance to resolve maximally before resuming the treatments, if necessary. Most often, a patient will experience 80% improvement in the leg vein areas with three or four treatments.

Q: What types of complications can be seen with sclerotherapy treatments?

A: Most commonly (besides a little "pricking" sensation at the site of the tiny needle sticks), we see some minor clots forming in the treated vessels. This will often appear as a darker vessel that seems to be filled with blood. It is. That's the clot that forms in some of the larger vessels, as the body forms a fibrous "cord" which is cleaned up systematically by the white blood cells in the area, resulting in complete resolution of the target vein. We frequently make a tiny, nearly invisible stab wound into these vein/clot areas, and express the clot right out to the surface with a cotton swab. If this is done to clotted areas, the healing and reattainment of a normal-appearing area is much more rapid.

Another frequently occurring problem is the appearance of tannish-brown pigment in the treated areas, as the veins begin to resolve. This is actually a temporary "tattoo" or "rust stain," which comes from the deposition of blood pigments and iron into the skin surrounding the treated vessels. It's slow to resolve, but will go away in almost every case, with a little watchful waiting. Regardless, the slight brownish stains that can result from sclerotherapy are really much more agreeable than the red spider-type veins that were there prior to treatment.

Q: What about ulceration? My doctor doesn't have aethoxysclerol (EOS, which you said doesn't usually cause sores in the areas of injection), and I'm afraid that using the strong salt solution will leave white scars on my legs in the areas of the injections. What do you think?

A: You are correct that ulcerative sores occur much more frequently with saline (salt solution) than with EOS. EOS is the stuff almost all modern sclerotherapists use for the tiniest of vessels, and when they are just learning the new technique. But if your doctor uses strong salt solution, he will probably have on hand a syringe of physiologic saline (that never causes ulcerative sores), which he can inject into any areas where he suspects an inadvertent spillage of strong saline under the epidermis. Dilution of the stronger salt solution with the milder, nonirritating solution will almost always protect the skin from necrosis (cell death, producing an ulcer and a subsequent scar).

Q: Will I know if spillage of hypertonic saline (HS, the strong salt solution) occurs in my skin?

A: Usually you will recognize a burning sensation, to which you should alert your dermatologist. In fact, you should feel a little cramping of the leg muscles when HS is injected, but any change in character of this or any other pain that occurs when the injections are done should be brought to the attention of your doctor immediately, so that he may dilute out the salt solution. This is very important. Even small extravasations (spills within the skin, outside the vein) can occasionally cause significant marks on the skin, so early notification will prevent problems.

Q: Can you be allergic to HS?

A: No. This has not been recorded.

Q: How about to EOS?

A: While true allergy to EOS is extremely rare, it does occasionally happen, and your doctor must be prepared for it. He'll have adrenalin, cortisone, and oxygen on hand, in case you have any serious distress with EOS. This is an extremely rare event, but it has happened.

Q: I recently traveled to a large city, in which I saw whole buildings labeled "Sclerotherapy Clinic"! I didn't see any advertisements for the doctor in charge, but he was a dermatologist. Is this a safe setting in which to get sclerotherapy injections for my painful veins?

A: That whole practices are devoted to sclerotherapy attests to the scope of the problem of ugly leg veins in women. Most of the dermatologists who do sclerotherapy do indeed maintain active practices of general dermatology also—I've yet to meet a highly trained dermatologist who would risk getting rusty in his general dermatology while devoting all his time to the performance of this one procedure. Even Dr. David Duffy, the person widely considered to be the world's expert in the technique of sclerotherapy, still sees many general dermatology patients in his practice as well as those seeking cosmetic procedures such as sclerotherapy. But the procedure is so successful and so very popular that a skilled practitioner can quickly fill his working day with vein patients if he chooses to.

Cautions about whole "clinics" for sclerotherapy? I would advise patients seeking care at such facilities to check out the credentials of the operator extremely thoroughly. Ask about educational background, specialty board acceptance, numbers of patients injected by the doctor, and so forth. Does the doctor himself do the injections? This is a technique which *can*, indeed, be taught to a skilled nurse, and patients often get a reduced rate for their sessions if treated by the nurse for the easier veins, and by the doctor in several sessions for the extremely small veins. Ask about this—you could get a very good deal, but you need to confirm the training of each and every person who will be doing the procedure. And you should never let your veins be injected without the doctor right on the premises!

13

Having the Hair
You've Always Wanted

*For every dollar spent in the treatment of
disease, there are $10 spent on quackery.*
—Albert M. Kligman, MD

*There is more felicity on the far side of
baldness than young men can possibly
imagine.*
—Logan Pearsall Smith

I thought long and hard about our concepts of aging before
including a chapter on hair loss for men *and* women. But
there were many questions to consider. Is hair loss in
women a severe enough problem to be included here? Is
there really anything we can *do* about it? Do enough women
even *have* hair loss to warrant addition of this chapter?

I answered these questions for myself by thinking of my
many patients (male *and* female) with hair loss, and how
they really *feel* about it. A middle-aged woman just passing menopause provided the impetus to include a chapter
on hair loss. Sandra came into my office one morning
practically distraught over her hair. As I approached her,
it was easy to see she wore a wig. She surprised me when
she ripped it off suddenly and said, "There! You can see
the problem! Now *help* me!" A problem for sure. Sandra's
hair was so thin that it barely covered her scalp. And it

was clearly what we call "female pattern" hair loss, in that it affected mainly the top of the scalp and front sides of the hairline.

She told a tearful tale of her recent years of hair loss, and the many physical exams and laboratory workups she had been through to try to find a cause—but none was discovered. It was, on talking to her, a classic case of female pattern loss. But what struck me so hard was the *amount* of anguish women like Sandra go through with hair loss. Society puts such a heavy premium on the beautiful hair of women that even temporary hair loss, like that suffered during chemotherapy, can be a life-ruining process. You can imagine the pain of the threat of permanent hair loss.

So I've included this chapter for those women, some 15%–20% in my practice, who do have some genetic loss as they age. And I've included it so that all other women who read this book will be able to offer some logical, scientific alternatives to their *husbands* as well. I would encourage them, as they read through this chapter, to *tell* their husbands (who, of course, have a *much* higher incidence of hair loss) that something now *can* be done. They no longer have to pursue the gimmicks they hear about on TV.

Women should also be aware that although the treatments I'll mention in this chapter *do* work, they are not yet FDA-approved for women's hair loss—a fact that seems very strange to me. And certainly, *no* prescription medicine (even *topically applied* ones) should be used during pregnancy unless approved by the obstetrician. We know of no problems in this regard involving Rogaine, but nobody ever wants to discover one, either.

Also be aware that many other factors play a role in hair loss for women. Among these are endocrinological (hormonal) problems, which can be quite difficult to work up. Your dermatologist will assist you in elucidating a cause for your hair loss and/or referring you to a competent endocrinologist for a complete evaluation.

Women will want to read this chapter for themselves and for their mates, who may not have discovered its recommendations on their own. I would encourage women whose husbands have a problem with hair loss to send them to a dermatologist as soon as possible—because for both sexes, time is of the essence!

The Magnitude of the Problem

A friend of mine sat down in the barber's chair one day to get what little hair he had left trimmed.

"How do you want this cut?" asked the barber, courteously.

My friend thought a moment, ran his hand over his thinning pate, and replied, "Thicker!"

The barber laughed, but neither my friend nor the millions of men losing hair would consider it much of a joke. For them, every day is a time of counting the hairs that fall into the tub or the shower (many men actually do!). And amazingly, at least in my private practice observations, worries are much more prevalent about hair loss than about almost any other skin condition affecting men. Only premalignant sunspots top hair loss in frequency of complaints in the private practice of dermatology.

Regretfully, many men think that asking a doctor about it is "unmacho," "unmasculine," or "unworthy" of a dermatologist's time, but that's just not true. That attitude ignores the fact that a dermatologist is a specialist involved with treating the skin, nails, and *hair*! And frankly, when *you* are concerned enough about a problem to even consider it, that's the time that you should let him consider it too. I've always maintained that there are no stupid questions—just (occasionally) some stupid answers. In short, if you've ever been concerned about your hair loss, it's valid to talk to your dermatologist about it. You'll be surprised—he'll be concerned, and there *are* ways to help that you may never have even *suspected*.

Factors in Male Pattern Hair Loss

To understand why my buddy, and millions of other men, are losing hair, you must understand the three components of what is commonly called "male pattern hair loss," or "male pattern alopecia," or, most properly, "androgenetic alopecia" (AGA). All these terms mean essentially the same thing, but it's the latter one that is most definitive in its description of what is actually happening in men's scalps.

First and foremost, a man must have been born into the right (or wrong!) family in order to develop male pattern loss. It's a *genetic* phenomenon. The gene that causes AGA is described as "autosomal dominant with incomplete penetrance." That means three things (put simply):

1. The gene for this trait is found on the autosomes, the nonsex chromosomes in each and every cell in the body.

2. In males, only one gene is necessary for expression (visible evidence of hair loss) of the trait.

3. Although "autosomal dominance" would *suggest* to scientists that if only the male had the gene, 50% of the couple's offspring would have visible hair loss, in fact somewhat less than 50% end up with the disease. As yet, no one has adequately explained why this is so.

You'd be amazed at the myths that abound about the origins of the hair loss trait. Take Larry, for instance, a young man with fairly intense AGA. "I just can't understand why I'm losing hair, Dr. Bark!" he exclaimed. "None of the males on my mother's side of the family have any hair loss. Where'd I get it?"

"What's your father and his father's hair pattern? And how about your paternal uncles?"

"Oh, well, my dad and his brothers are almost *cue balls*," laughed Larry, "but everybody knows you don't get it from your dad's side of the family—isn't that right?"

Youth Alert!

Hats and helmets, even tight ones, have nothing to do with male pattern hair loss.

"Hardly," I said examining what was left of his thinning locks. What I had to tell Larry was quite a shock to him. He really believed that this was a disease for which mothers are responsible. The fact is, the gene passes down on *both* sides of the family. That's proof of the gene's presence on the autosomes and not the sex chromosomes.

But sometimes the myths are multiple. Larry insisted that even if that were true, *he* shouldn't have inherited the condition, because "everybody knows that it skips every other generation, doesn't it?" Sorry, wrong again. There's no truth at all that male pattern hair loss "skips" every other generation. It skips only those who don't have all three factors necessary for its appearance, and for no other reasons. If you stop and think about it, we all know families in whom there are two or more, if not *many*, consecutive generations with male pattern loss. I've tried to track down the origin of that piece of medical folklore, but have never been successful (incidentally, if you happen to know, write me, will you?).

An easier one to track is the one about wearing football helmets or hats as a cause of AGA. Around the time young men are engaged in high school football, they also develop the hormones necessary to cause the loss of hair, assuming they have the hair loss genetic material. That's why young kids think the helmets cause the loss—because it's *temporally* related (occurs at the same approximate time), that's all, not because the helmet causes a lack of circulation and subsequent loss.

And that brings up the *second* factor in AGA, *age*. You must reach the right age to develop the hormones we talked about above. On the other hand, you've never seen a 10-

---

Youth Alert!

You must have all three factors to show male pattern hair loss (AGA): inheritance, age, and hormones.

---

year-old boy with AGA, thus proving the right age must be attained before onset of the problem.

The *third* factor necessary to develop AGA is *hormones*, made by the male testes, and to a small extent in the adrenal glands (that's why the Bald Persons of America's motto is, "You can waste your male hormones on growing hair if you want to, but not me!").

The one hormone most responsible for hair loss is called DHT (*di*hydro*t*estosterone), a derivative of the male hormone testosterone which is tens of times more potent in causing hair loss than testosterone itself. It causes miniaturization of the normal, thick, adult-looking hairs that we all want to keep on our scalps. The proof of its relationship to baldness is that it is present in much higher concentrations in the cells of hair follicles in the front of the scalp of balding men than in nonbalding men.

Bald Men Are *Not* Bald!

Note that I said "miniaturization" of the hairs. It's always been fascinating to me that the bald are really not actually bald. Their hair-making apparatus has simply followed

---

Youth Alert!

Daily washing is vital in slowing the loss of hair in AGA. Use a good de-oiling shampoo, like Ionil Plus, and you may, just by this method alone, slow your loss tremendously!

---

its genetic program for this particular time in the man's life and caused the follicles to regress in size and to grow very tiny, so that the hairs made now are nearly invisible. But you can see them if you try—get a strong magnifying glass sometime and take a look at a "balding" scalp. You, too, will be amazed to see how tiny the hairs are—*thousands* of them! A veritable forest! And it's exactly those hairs at which the newer chemical methods of hair regrowth are directed. Certainly, some gradual loss of follicles occurs just as a result of senescence, but most men still have most of them. More about this later.

The normal human body has about 5 million hairs, with 1 million of those on the neck and head, and about 100,000 of that million on the scalp itself (yes, someone *did* actually sit down at a microscope and *count* them!). The hairs on the scalp grow about 0.37 millimeters per day, and can reach lengths of 50 centimeters or more before cycling to the resting phase and dropping out. Some fantastic exceptions to these numbers exist, however, and one fellow actually willed his 28-*foot* beard to the Smithsonian!

Quack Treatments

My mentor in dermatology once told me that if we looked around for fake, unethical methods for treating AGA, we would find about as many of them as there are patients to be treated! After years and years of dealing with men desperate to keep the hair they had, I can attest to the truth of *that* statement. And discouragingly, every time we get a hint of something new actually *working* in AGA, someone either comes along and discovers a problem with it, or the legitimate interest in the substance or technique is diluted by the attempt of every cosmetic company to "jump on the bandwagon" and claim they have something just as good in one or more of their products, which doesn't require a prescription or "an expensive trip to the doctor."

Youth Alert!

*So you're growing less and less hair these days?
Beware! There are thousands of charlatans who
would like to scalp you as well.*

Of course, it's a problem not only in the treatment of AGA but in the case of the entire Retin-A story, too.

What, then, is the effect of treatments such as massages, which are meant to "stimulate circulation" in the scalp? Is there any place for such techniques in hair loss? Not unless you're really into throwing your money away. And there are a lot better and more enjoyable ways to do that. Many of us dermatologists actually believe those massages are injurious to the appearance, by rubbing out or pulling out hair follicles just now cycling into the resting phase, and normally due to stay in the scalp for several more months. The bottom line here is: Why massage them and pull them out *early*?

How about the many hundreds of quacks and hucksters on television who hawk their products to an unsuspecting public? Isn't there a law to stop such misrepresentation? Unfortunately not. It's really a disgusting situation—P. T. Barnum would have loved every minute of it. In Lexington we have two or three half-hour cable TV shows a week all about some crazy, bogus hair restorer that's guaranteed to grow hair "or your money back." Of course, *none* of them work, but you'd be surprised at how many testimonials they scare up about the magic results obtained on their "new system." I'm always amazed at how many of the male promoters of these products are themselves extremely thin of hair, if not actually bald. Wouldn't you think, if it was such a great product, that they'd latch onto it and actually use some of it themselves? Does that tell you anything?

And the prices! It's not uncommon to see prices in the neighborhood of $60–$80 for a two-month "supply." Usually, when you receive these products, they consist of a simple shampoo, sometimes gunked up with some complicating ingredients like jojoba oil, aloe vera, braised oil of African rhino horn, or some other useless chemicals. Some even contain elements of wheat germ oil, which itself can sometimes encourage even more loss! If you figure that some of these shows, aired nationwide on cable, have about $37,000 or more in expenses *per hour*, they must be selling enough of these useless potions to sink a battleship! But then, the useless ingredients are worth only a few cents per bottle. Talk about profit margins!

In practice, what these companies do is devise a product and convince several "camera ready" victims to "tell their stories" on tape, and then they bicycle these tapes around the country to all the major markets and play them continually (sometimes once per *day*!) until orders coming into their central facility taper off. Then the tapes are sent on to another market. Sometimes, the station running the tapes won't even charge for the airtime—instead, they take a percentage cut on what new customers order.

Naturally, none of the stuff they sell is any better than commonly available over-the-counter shampoos and conditioners, even though they tell you it's the greatest thing since sliced bread. Interestingly, even though most of these charlatans are just ordinary Joes who worked a new idea for bilking the public, there seems to be no lack of "doctor figures" on the stages with them, sometimes in lab coats, even, touting the "medical benefits" of the new system. Often, they'll use the words "dermatologist approved," or "doctor tested." Hokum. Pure and simple. Where's the FDA when we need 'em?

I watched one of these shows with great interest just a few months ago. It purported to have the final answer to hair loss in men, a chemical that was, they announced, investigated and approved by two renowned dermatolo-

━━━━━ *Youth Alert!* ━━━━━

Don't be fooled by claims that a product is "hypoallergenic," or "doctor approved." These terms can apply to some of the worst junk on the market today.

gists. I wondered about this, because I had never heard of either of them, nor had I heard of their "miracle chemical cure" for AGA. So I decided to call their bluff. Since they claimed that major medical journals had reported the findings of the investigating doctors in recent years, I logged on to "PaperChase," a service that accesses the National Library of Medicine's literature file of over 3 *million* articles written in the last 20 years, concerning each and every facet of medicine. I spent hours doing a thorough literature search, and *not a single one* of those 3 million articles even *mentioned* the ingredient. Now *that's* just how accurate such statements are. Ethical, effective products are investigated and reported in the ethical, refereed journals of medicine and science. It's as simple as that.

But stories about products like this are not hard to find. That just shows how resilient is human hope, especially with regard to what I call "cosmosocial" skin problems—problems which, although commonly considered cosmetic, are extremely important in our daily social interaction with our colleagues, friends, and acquaintances. Many people, in fact *thousands*, will rush to their checkbooks for any new hope of a cure for hair loss. That's just how much importance we attach to it.

Save your money! And think of this: With that same amount of money, you probably could have had a consultation with an excellent dermatologist and could have received a prescription for the topical mixture I'll tell you about shortly.

How *Dermatologists* Treat Hair Loss

What actually *can* be done for male pattern alopecia? Plenty! Realize that I am *not* talking "cure" here. Nobody has a cure yet for this condition, and anybody who tells you he *does* (with the possible exception of hair transplants and scalp reduction surgery, to be discussed later) is lying to you.

First, let me remind you of the important function daily washing plays in the retarding of male pattern hair loss. Remember the superpowerful hormone DHT we mentioned earlier? This substance, besides being tightly bound to receptors inside the cytoplasm of the cells, is found in high concentrations in the sebum, and is secreted with this oil onto the surface of the scalp. There it lies on the surface of the skin, and is *re*absorbed into the scalp and recycled into the hair follicle cells, where it causes yet *more* loss! This is a tremendous opportunity to interdict the supply of this hair loss hormone, so that loss may be slowed.

Will you hurt your hair by washing it as often as once a day? Won't that make it dead, lifeless, dry? No, washing hair as often as once a day will not hurt it, except in the case where it has already been damaged by chemical treatment for bleaching, permanents, and so on. Dead? Lifeless? Your hair is already dead! There's never been a living hair in the history of the human race. So you can't kill what's already dead! In practice, what is often meant by this expression is that the hair will be "flyaway," or static-laden, which makes its feel disagreeable. You can rid yourself of that feel just by using a great conditioner (like the "medical" conditioner, Ionil Rinse, which many dermatologists advise for their patients).

What should a man do if he starts to notice hair loss? The worst thing he can do is sit around and worry about it without dermatologic consultation. Assuming he has accepted the fact that he has a real and valid problem that

====== *Youth Alert!* ======

Washing the hair once daily will remove DHT from the scalp, slowing down hair loss. For this daily wash, use a good de-oiling shampoo, like Ionil Plus (Owen Company).

is not going to go away, and may, in fact, get progressively worse, he can turn to the new chemical methods to prevent further loss and perhaps restore some of what has fallen. But time is critical here. The drugs I'll be telling you about work best the sooner the treatment is begun. To sit around and worry about it or to pursue the many quack remedies promoted on TV and in popular magazines without *doing* something is craziness in its finest form, because hair loss is most treatable at the outset, and less and less treatable with the passage of time.

The Rogaine (Minoxidil) Story

That brings us to the story of minoxidil, one of the most fascinating tales of discovery in all of dermatology. Physicians who initially used the anti-hypertensive (anti–high blood pressure) medication minoxidil noticed a peculiar side effect. Some of the patients who took it developed excess hair growth in some really unusual places, like the face and the forehead. In fact, some of these patients, who obviously couldn't give up the medicine because of its

====== *Youth Alert!* ======

Losing hair? Don't tarry! The sooner you start medicine for your hair loss, the greater the chance it'll work. Best time? The teens. Worst time? After age 40.

> ## ═══ *Youth Alert!* ═══
>
> *Pharmacist-prepared topical minoxidil (as opposed to that prepared by the Upjohn Company, which, as of August 1988 is approved) is not FDA-approved for use in male pattern baldness. But keep in mind that FDA-unapproved does not mean ineffective.*

salutary effect on high blood pressure, actually began to shave their foreheads and faces to keep down the obvious hair growth. It was a very disturbing side effect indeed, especially for the women who used the medicine!

But as so often occurs, a little serendipity supplemented the science in this scenario. Dermatologists who consulted with their colleagues about this strange side effect wondered whether it couldn't somehow be used to combat one of their most common office complaints, and one of the most difficult to treat, male pattern loss. They reasoned that if the drug could be put into a lotion and rubbed onto the skin, perhaps some of the hairs could be made to return. Sure enough, it worked! Or rather, I should say, it worked in some patients and not in others.

The maker of minoxidil, Upjohn, started sponsoring nationwide tests that were intended to lead toward approval and release of this medication under the aegis of the FDA. Tests conducted in more than 3,500 patient volunteers over several years showed up to 30% of the patients using minoxidil actually got a return of at least some of the "terminal" (mature, visible) dark brown or black hairs that we were all intended to have. So they sought approval from the Dermatology Panel of the FDA, a group consisting of some of the most respected skin researchers in this country.

That panel approved the compound for release, although they said that, in their opinion, only approximately one-seventh of the patients actually *regrew* hair, but many, if not most, of the others seemed to hold on to what they had. The proposal for release went to the FDA in general, which declined to release it at that time, demanding more and more clinical trials to prove its salutary effect, until August 1988, when the final approval came for the sale of the medicine. It was the step that many balding men were waiting for.

For many, especially the balding men of this country, that would have been enough—but not for the FDA. They required the *name* of the prescription product be changed, from "Regaine" to "Rogaine," because it was felt the former implied a "promise" that hair would regrow. That was somewhat ridiculous, I'd say, in light of the number of products that promise everything from "Gee, Your Hair Smells Terrific!" to "Suave," and to my knowledge, none of those promises have ever been proven to occur either. It just meant that a lot of "o's" would be pasted over a lot of "e's," that's all.

Rumor had it that Upjohn had a huge warehouse full of the compound in Canada (where it has been approved for use for some time) just waiting for the word from the FDA to be moved into this country. Upjohn even erected one of the most advanced pharmaceutical production facilities ever designed, just to meet the expected demand for this medication. Obviously, their marketing studies showed that men would be beating down the door to get the stuff, and we dermatologists were very excited about the possibility of finally being able to write a prescription for the medicine in its FDA-approved form.

But that's hardly the end of the story. Minoxidil is, by itself, effective in reversing some AGA, but at the 1987 American Academy of Dermatology meeting, new and important studies were released that showed minoxidil *much* more effective if *combined with Retin-A*! How much more effective? Well, suffice it to say that it's tremendously more effective—some say as many as *50%* of the users of the mixture will *regain* hair (good *terminal* hair), and most of the rest will *keep* the hair they have! For the balding men of this country, *that's* effective.

What's the hitch in all this? Upjohn has not yet obtained permission to market any combination drugs containing minoxidil *and* Retin-A. They claimed in one video conference I attended that such a combination would possibly cause increased absorption of the minoxidil, since increased penetration of chemicals into the skin is one of the effects researchers have noted with Retin-A, although I've used this combination in hundreds of patients over the last 18 months and have noted not one single adverse effect. That's not a scientific proof of effectiveness, certainly, just a statement of my own experiences with this drug. Currently, studies of this very combination are ongoing in a number of major dermatologic centers in this country to determine formally its safety and efficacy. Interestingly, penetration of the minoxidil must not be the whole story, since Retin-A by itself, applied to the scalps of balding men, will cause some significant regrowth of hair!

Application of the Medicine

Upjohn supplies three different applicators with each unit of Rogaine: a sprayer for larger areas, a dauber for tiny areas, and an extended spray attachment for getting into hairy areas easily, which work very nicely. Upjohn recommends that you treat the entire top of the head, though, because each of their metered attachments delivers one cubic centimeter (cc) of the liquid if used exactly as directed, and that's what they recommend will cover the entire top of the scalp.

Please also keep in mind that this medicine is not to be applied to a diseased scalp (psoriasis, severe seborrheic dermatitis, folliculitis, and others), nor to a scalp irritated by treatments for other conditions. If these are present, they must be treated first; then the Rogaine treatments can be started.

Frequency of application is critical to the success of any topical treatment. As a rule, it's necessary to treat the skin twice daily so that the medicine soaks in to the necessary area of involvement. This is true of other topicals, such as antibiotics used in acne and many cortisone medications used in other skin diseases. So use it twice daily, just as directed by your dermatologist. Investigators saw a significant drop in effectiveness when patients treated themselves less than twice daily. And contrarily, *no* greater effect was seen if the medicine was used *more* often than twice a day—in fact, the chances of adverse consequences are greater when the frequency is increased, as you'd expect.

How long must you treat? The answer to this question is based on a very simple physiological fact of hair growth: Hairs grow a long time (often 2–10 *years*) and rest a short time (usually 3–4 months). But the fact that that "short" resting phase time, in human hair, *does* last for a matter of months means you can't expect the minoxidil to work much before 6–8 months, and it's probably wiser to do as I tell my patients to do—count on using the medicine for a full year to confirm whether or not it's doing you any good.

I realize that at $40–$50 per month, I'm asking you to commit to quite an investment, but we know that Rogaine will help a vast number of men, so I'd recommend it heartily for any man with AGA. The nice fact is, even in those men in whom Rogaine doesn't actually *regrow* hair, it *can* help hang on to what they have! That has to be worth the "price of admission," for most men, at least!

Insurance Coverage for Rogaine?

Can you get your health insurance plan to pay for this prescription? I can't guarantee anything in this regard, but I can tell you this: *Many* of my hair loss patients tell me that they *do* get reimbursed for this medicine from their insurance companies. It falls into a new and rather nebulous category of medicine that the illustrious Dr. Albert

Kligman calls "cosmeceuticals," which the insurance companies are scrutinizing much more closely.

I make no recommendation whatsoever to patients on whether to submit such claims, but I repeat that many have told me their insurance plans do cover the medicine, especially now that it has been released for hair growth by the FDA. The same question, you'll remember from the Retin-A chapters, arises for that medicine (and collagen too), and the same answer applies. We're fast approaching a whole new era in medicine, in which drugs that really do work for medico-cosmetic indications are being rapidly developed. That means insurance companies are developing new guidelines for the reimbursement of patients for these drugs.

Can you *stop* using minoxidil if it works for you? Will all your hair fall out if you do? The answers to these all-important questions are not fully determined yet, but from what we know about preliminary use of this medicine in male pattern loss, you probably will lose all the ground you've gained if you stop the medicine. And the loss will usually start about two weeks after stopping the medicine. Sad but true—you'll need to realize this and be ready to commit to possibly a lifetime of using the medicine if it *does*, in fact, work for you.

What if you're away on a trip and forget to take your medicine? In a word, *don't*! You may, it's thought, miss two to four days of Rogaine with no excess loss, but anything longer than that and you're risking looking quite a bit different on your return home than when you left! And then, the worst part of stopping Rogaine is that it'll take you another hair cycle and more months to get it all back again.

Is it worth all that? Only you can make that decision, but my own word of advice for men with hair loss is *go for it*! Do all you can to stay young-looking, good-looking, and comfortable as long as humanly possible. As they say, this is the real thing, not practice, so you might as well look as good as you can for the time you've got!

Other Alternatives for Hair Replacement

But what if medicines and daily shampooing don't work to retard your loss and grow you new hair? There are many alternatives right now, and new ones are arising all the time. What I'm trying to say here is that almost every man who really wants to look as if he has never lost hair can do exactly that, under the guidance of the proper experts. Let's talk about some advanced surgical alternatives to baldness.

Transplants

Hair transplantation has been around since the early 1950s, pioneered and perfected by dermatologist Dr. Norman Orentreich in 1955, who invented the tiny skin punches that make this technique so successful.

It has long been a mystery why hairs around the sides of the scalp remain, when those in front, the "monk's cap" toward the back of the scalp, and the large field of scalp between them fall out so readily in men who have the genes for hair loss. One would think that all the cells of the scalp would contain the same genetic material, and that the hormones, which circulate equally in all areas, should cause loss equally in all areas too. But we all know that's not what happens. We have all seen hundreds of men with a good growth of hair around the edges of the scalp, and virtually none whatsoever (except the micro-fine miniature vellus hairs I mentioned earlier) on the top of the scalp (the vertex). So something must happen to those hair production cells that makes them more sensitive to male hormone. That something is called differentiation.

Differentiation basically refers to the ability of some cells in the body to express themselves differently as they develop. We see innumerable examples of this in every

=== *Youth Alert!* ===

The genetic origin of AGA is amply proven by observing hair loss after transplantation. Because the donor hairs came from the sides of the scalp, they are not nearly as susceptible to loss. In effect, that means those transplanted hairs will remain in the scalp until the side hairs fall out! And that usually never happens!

organism. Some cells, despite identical genetic material at birth, make teeth instead of toenails, or ears instead of kidneys. In a similar manner, the expression of "hairiness" is determined by that same variable factor. Some of the scalp cells, like those around the edges, are not as responsive to DHT hormone as are those on the top of the scalp in the traditional baldness areas.

The really wonderful thing about differentiation is that it is permanent for hair follicles. That is, once the scalp follicle cells have been determined to be constant hair producers, even in the face of DHT, they *remain* hair producers for nearly a person's whole life. What does all this mean? It means that if you have a transplant from the sides of the scalp to the balding area, those hairs will keep growing (after an initial shocklike fallout period) for as long as the donor site retains *its* hairs. At first, surgeons didn't know this fact, and tried hair transplantation a few times to see if, in fact, those transplanted hairs would fall right out like their neighbors had. Thankfully, they did not. (Well, that's not exactly true. They *did* fall out at first, due to the shock of the surgery, but promptly regrew.) And that opened the door to all the wonderful hair transplant operations we've seen since those early days.

Refinements of technique in transplanting hairs have come steadily. As the operation is now done, small plugs of hair-bearing skin are taken from the sides of the scalp and are inserted into holes made with a similar punch in

---

Youth Alert!

All newly planted hairs do fall out, but they promptly regrow.

---

the hairless areas. These plugs heal and start to grow hair within a few short weeks.

This conventional transplant procedure has several drawbacks. The biggest of these is the fact the transplant *is*, in fact, done in plugs. That means there has been a lot of objection to the "corn row" effect noticed by many transplantees. This is especially noticeable around the edges of the transplanted area—essentially, it is a very visible, cut off–looking hairline, which informs everyone who looks at the patient that he has undergone a transplant.

The other frequent complication of hair transplantation surgery is that when the hairs grow out, they seem to be aiming in an unnatural direction. This is largely a matter of finding a very *experienced* surgeon, who understands the development and construction of a transplanted hairline. Most surgeons who do the operation frequently are extremely aware of this, and will align the plugs correctly to produce a hairline that looks as natural as possible.

The first problem is much more difficult to solve. A hairline, you should understand, is just that, a *line*! And that almost always looks unnatural, because in life, the hairline is really an *area*, where the hair gradually thins to apparent hairlessness. This has been a tough nut to crack, until a revolutionary development occurred, called the micrograft transplant dilator.

Micrografts

The micrograft technique involves the transplanting of *individual hairs* into tiny holes made by a rodlike instru-

---

Youth Alert!

Remember that the most important part of the transplant is the hairline.

---

ment at the front hairline area. Then grafts of *one hair each* are meticulously harvested from the edges of the regularly done graft plugs. These are inserted one at a time in a random fashion along the hairline area to give a natural, *blended* appearance to the front limits of the transplant.

Some of the photos of the hairline produced by this technique are nothing short of spectacular. If you or any member of your family or any male acquaintance are contemplating a hair transplant, you owe it to yourself to see the beautiful photographs in the *Journal of Dermatologic Surgery and Oncology*, March 1988, by the physician who perfected this technique in North America, Dr. Emanuel Marritt. Dr. Marritt, clinical instructor in hair transplantation in the Department of Otolaryngology, Head and Neck Surgery at the University of Colorado School of Medicine, Denver, published his findings and technique for all physicians to see. His photographs of the results of this technique are nothing short of miraculous.

Dr. Marritt begins the micrograft sessions during the very first transplant session (by unnoticeably taking a few hairs from the edges of each graft plug), and continues them right through the fourth session, which is usually the final one in his transplant program. If need be, he will see patients on subsequent occasions to implant more single hairs with the micrograft technique. He has even refined this latter technique to a sort of "mass grafting" of single hairs to smooth out and even the hairline. This is truly a transplant that looks as if the recipient had been born

---

═══ *Youth Alert!* ═══

The most important part of your initial visit with the transplant surgeon is to evaluate his photographs, which should be of excellent quality.

---

with it! If you want more information on his fabulous technique, just call 303-694-9371, or write him at:

> Dr. Emanuel Marritt
> The Quadrant
> 5445 DTC Parkway, Suite 1015
> Englewood, CO 80111

His success is truly remarkable. And while it is obvious that Dr. Marritt himself could not micrograft every man with AGA who reads this book, he certainly does have suggestions on the most important information to request when discussing a transplant.

Here, in abbreviated form, is his chief advice to prospective transplantees:

The single most important criterion for evaluating the skill and expertise of a hair transplant surgeon is the careful examination of his before-and-after photographs. It is the most reliable indicator of the results that you, the prospective patient, can expect on your own head.

When evaluating photographs, *never* trust any pictures that are blurry Polaroids, taken from too far away, under- or over-exposed (too light or too dark), or photos that attempt to hide the hairline by combing the hair forward or concealing the hairline with the curls of a perm. Remember, you do not want to see the hairline at its styled *best*. You want to see it at its *worst*. Therefore, always *insist* on clear, 35mm quality, color photographs, taken from the part side with a visible comb in the picture that combs the hair back to reveal (not conceal) the hairline. The technique of combing the hair backward assures you that the hair you see *on* the forehead is actually growing *from* the forehead, and not being combed forward from the side fringe.

Furthermore, make sure that the photographs demonstrate a series of *progressive* close-up photography to convince you that the extreme final close-up of the hairline (last picture) actually belongs to the same patient as the one in the first picture.

Insist on seeing photographs of patients with dark hair and light skin. This difficult color combination provides for maximum contrast of hair and skin and most accurately reflects the skill of the surgeon. A poorly performed transplant may photograph as an acceptable result in patients who have the natural camouflaging combinations of blond, red, or gray hair and ruddy complexion.

Moreover, don't be ashamed to ask the surgeon if the photographs that he is showing you are of his own patients and not from a text or medical article. Finally, if you still have any lingering doubts, ask to visit with and talk to one or two of his completed patients. Patients who are happy with their result are more than willing to share their experience with another "bald brother," so be wary if the surgeon refuses to let you see photographs or patients, while claiming "patient confidentiality."

Remember, you can be respectful but also assertive. This is, after all, *your* bald head, and you are going to stare at the finished product each and every morning for the rest of your life as you shave, wash, and brush your teeth. You have a right to have hair that looks like a *forest*, not an *apple orchard*!

That just about says it all. There is no doubt in my mind at all that this is the finest hair transplant procedure available on this planet.

Scalp Reduction Surgery

Not everyone's hair loss problem is identical, and not every replacement technique or medical treatment would or even should be the same. Many variations of the corrective techniques I recommend in this chapter are available, and it's up to you to question your doctor to see which is most appropriate in your individual case.

One of the most dramatic kinds of surgery for this problem is called scalp reduction surgery. In this advanced technique, a skilled transplant surgeon can actually cut out all or part of a man's bald spot! Sounds incredible, doesn't it? But this revolutionary technique, when combined with one called "tissue expansion," can greatly reduce the size of the area that may have to receive transplants in the future.

As with all the other techniques we've discussed, scalp reduction has a downside as well. Scarring is a problem, as is occasional temporary hair loss around the edges of the surgical site, but this is a very valuable method in those for whom it was designed.

Scalp Flaps

Another surgical technique involves the rotation of hair-bearing areas of skin into the areas that are bald. This is not really a transplant, since the hair-bearing skin that is rotated into the hairless area is never really *separated* from the donor area, but is a *movement* of hairy skin to cover a balding spot.

Again, scarring is sometimes a problem, but the rotated flaps of hairy skin and the adjacent hairy areas will often cover this sufficiently. Both this method and scalp reduction surgery are serious procedures which can occasionally result in excessive bleeding and scarring, and, like *any* surgical procedure, they are not to be approached lightly.

An Unacceptable Surgical Technique

Besides the many quack gimmicks on the market to "make hair grow," some dubious surgical techniques are promoted as well. The most damaging to the scalp is one called "fiber implantation," which was popular up until a few years ago. In this technique, strings of suturelike material were passed underneath the scalp skin and secured at the other side of the scalp, where hairlike clumps of material were attached. Often, the body was smart enough to react to the implanted material and eject it from the skin, but the charlatans who performed this procedure on thousands of men defeated the body's own protective mechanism by *tying knots* in the implanted fibers! In many patients this caused extraordinary scarring and infection in the scalp skin. Many victims of fiber implantation will carry the scars for life, and have no practical solution to their AGA except extensive, expensive plastic surgery. It's a sad, sad story—one that I hope will never be repeated. I've treated a couple of these men myself in my office, and I've never seen a more miserable lot of triple losers: They've lost their hair, gained severe scars, and still have to go through the conventional transplant procedures if they expect to have good coverage. Sadly enough, because of the scarring, these are the men who *need* coverage by transplantation most. Bottom line? There's no free lunch in surgical hair replacement, and won't be for years to come.

Choosing a Surgeon

It should be obvious from the preceding horror story that you should choose your dermatologist or surgeon in a manner akin to picking a spouse—*very carefully*! It cannot be overstressed that you should receive a thorough consultation before making a decision. Make sure the surgeon has proper credentials, such as a *board certificate* from the American Academy of Dermatology, the American Society of Plastic and Reconstructive Surgeons Inc., or the American Board of Plastic Surgery.

Realize, though, that just about anyone with enough diligence can obtain certification from *some* official body, and that certification alone is not good enough. You should ask for patient references, so that you can actually talk to some of the surgeon's patients who have had the same operation he is proposing for you. And you should insist on seeing a *host* of photographs of patients who've had the operation.

If you learn one thing from this chapter on improving the look of your scalp, let it be this: If you skip these all-important steps in picking a suitable surgeon, you're taking your very skin into your hands. I certainly wouldn't claim you as one of the "students" of my program, that's for sure.

But done correctly, scalp surgery for hair replacement or relocation is a wonderfully successful and rewarding type of surgery to have, ranking right up there with cataract surgery in the elderly, and plastic surgery for birthmarks, scars, and wrinkles. Performed by a surgeon of concern and competence, these procedures will reward you every time you look into the mirror, probably for the rest of your life. Done incorrectly or in haste, that same mirror will make you curse the day you ever discovered such surgery was possible. In Chapter 10 I give recommendations about picking a plastic/cosmetic surgeon. Read that chapter carefully in light of what you've learned here about hair transplantation.

Commonly Asked Questions About AGA

Q: Is Rogaine safe?

A: Absolutely. In all the 3,500 patients tested so far, no serious adverse consequences have been found. And in over five years of use in the offices of private practitioners of dermatology, the same is true. About the most we see as a complication is irritation of the scalp.

Q: How long does the anagen (active growing phase) cycle last?

A: About a thousand days. This is highly variable, though, if you'll just look around at the normal population differences to prove this to yourself.

Q: Are there any clues as to how Rogaine actually works?

A: There are two current theories, neither of which has been proved, but work goes on to narrow down the possibilities.

The *direct* theory says that the medicine actually stimulates the very hair-making cells of the dermal papilla—that's the action center of hair production. The other theory, based on the clearly defined functions of minoxidil in hypertension, is that it acts like a vasodilator: It opens up the blood vessels inside the dermal papilla, causing greater amounts of oxygen and nutrients to grow more hair.

Q: Should I apply Rogaine to my entire scalp, since my dad had much more extensive loss than I do currently?

A: Absolutely! Anyone who uses this medicine should apply it to the entire top of the scalp, to prevent extension of the area of loss. Use the medicine exactly as suggested with one of the three applicators supplied with the treatment kit.

Q: Will my gray hair darken if I start to use Rogaine?

A: Yes, there is some evidence obtained informally in the scientific studies to suggest that some men do indeed regain some of their youthful color to their graying hairs. This is highly individual, however, and I certainly wouldn't count on it.

Q: Will an old man respond?

A: Not nearly as well, but there are some cases on record in which older men did beautifully on Rogaine. That again is highly individual, and really seems to depend on the number of hairs, even the tiny vellus or baby-fine hairs, that remain in the area prior to treatment with Rogaine. If there are a lot of hairs, then the chances of regrowing some hair are much higher. Again, no guarantees.

Q: Should I really try this stuff, or am I just delaying my transplant for a year or two to confirm that Rogaine will not help me?

A: I personally think everyone should try this medicine before seriously contemplating a transplant. However, let me put in a plug (so to speak) for transplants. This operation is one of the most proven and successful in all dermatology, and if your social situation demands faster restoration of your hair, like some of the congressmen, actors, and others who have had it done in the past, then I would go right ahead with it. Of course, these two treatments are not mutually exclusive. You can sign up for your hair transplant and still use Rogaine at the same time. That way, any thickening you get from the Rogaine will possibly decrease the need for further transplantation. The important effect of Rogaine use in transplant candidates is that the medicine really stops further loss in the majority of men, regardless of whether it makes your areas of loss look ape-like again.

Q: Any hints for how to tell when the liquid has reached all areas of the scalp?

A: One of the neatest tricks in using Rogaine is to store it in the freezer overnight before use (don't worry, it won't freeze, because the vehicle in which the minoxidil is mixed is like anti-freeze). Then when you apply the mixture, using whatever applicator you've chosen as best for you, you'll definitely feel the areas where the medicine hits your skin.

Q: What if my kids start losing hair like I did at age 13 or 14? Can we start it on them too?

A: Yes, the medicine does look safe for that population, but remember, you're putting your kids on a scalp medicine that they may not, then, be able to stop for the rest of their natural life! That decision has to be made very carefully with your physician, cooperating with your dermatologist. Anyway, the medicine does appear safe in that age group—it's just a question of whether you and they are ready for such a difficult, twice-a-day regimen of applying a topical medicine.

Q: Can I use hair tonics and regular shampoos with Rogaine therapy?

A: Yes, but make sure that when you apply the Rogaine, your scalp is dry. Wet scalps tend to dilute the medicine and stop it from working.

Q: How hard will it be to get hold of suitable patch test materials to test Rogaine, if I should become allergic to some component of it?

A: No problem with patch testing with Rogaine is expected, because the company supplies inquiring physicians with a free patch test kit with all the ingredients broken down for easy reference if any of the tests is positive.

Q: What happens at 12 months into the study of patients on Rogaine? Do they continue to improve?

A: It does indeed look like the maximum growth with Rogaine occurs in the first 12 months. After that, most men hit a plateau, showing a steady state for hair growth. After five years of use, most men retain their one-year hair counts, with a few sagging just below the improved number of hairs. We think the growth phase has been extended with the use of Rogaine, but some resting hairs are still seen, so that minimal loss continues, probably throughout life, even though Rogaine is being used.

Q: Is minoxidil safe to use in women, and especially, is it safe to use in pregnancy?

A: There is currently no approved indication for the use of Rogaine in women, despite the fact that many of them develop a condition known as "female pattern loss" in their 40s and 50s which could be helped by Rogaine—we just don't know the whole story about *everything* that it will help yet.

Q: Where can I get further information on Rogaine?

A: Call Upjohn's Rogaine Answer Line at 800-635-0655. There'll be someone there to answer all your questions, or else refer you to someone who can.

14

How to Avoid Itchy, Dry Skin

Ten percent of those over 70 have over 10 skin problems that need evaluation.

—*Albert M. Kligman, MD*

One of the most frequent problems I'm asked about is the dry skin associated with aging. No less than 40% of patients over 40 years old have some element of dryness, and many of them don't even realize why they may be itching, scaling, and flaking more as the years pass.

A Poorly Understood but Important Problem

Because of my extensive experience with this problem as a clinical dermatologist who treats it every day of his life, I've got some great *practical* tips that can really help you tremendously. Some of the tips you'll read here have been discussed briefly in other chapters, such as my favorite moisturizer recommendations and soap advice, but I thought that putting all this information in one place so you could refer to it easily would be helpful to you. Not that reversing your dry skin will really make you any younger—it won't. But it could make you a whole lot more comfortable as you go through the winters, whether or

Youth Alert!

No moisturizer or other over-the-counter product can ever reverse a single wrinkle on your face. All claims for anti-aging based on anything other than a sunscreen are pure hokum!

not you use Retin-A and all the other measures mentioned in this book.

Nobody, not even the most advanced clinical research-ers, seems to understand the real problem of dry skin. Oh sure, a few of us have been lucky enough to stumble onto the solutions, or find out how to treat it effectively from our respective mentors in dermatology, but for the most part, I find the actual day-to-day treatment of dry skin one of the least understood problems in modern derma-tology. And by my way of figuring, if *dermatologists* don't fully understand the magnitude and severity and *treat-ment* of the dry skin problem, trying to get help for this condition from your family doctor or other nondermatol-ogists is almost impossible.

Drying Out, Not Drying Up!

Here's the problem, pure and simple: We dry out with old age. And "old" doesn't have to mean *ancient*, either. But that statement, simple and straightforward as it is, would not be agreed upon by all the dermatology experts in the field of aging. Some say that the dead layer of the skin even gets *moister* with age! Preposterous! And few phy-sicians and dermatologists understand the role that too-frequent bathing plays in the cause and persistence of dry skin.

Let me give you this example of a patient with what I call dry skin, and see if you, as a layman, can tell me

---

Youth Alert!

Too-frequent bathing is one of the most severe causes of dry skin in the wintertime.

---

what's wrong. Sidney, age 62, has a real problem. He puts it this way: "Dr. Bark, every night when I take off my socks, I itch like nobody's business. I mean, this is such a nuisance that I shake the bed and wake my wife some nights!"

I asked Sid if he would take off his socks and show me his legs. As he pulled off his knee-high socks, the dust started flying! That's right, *dust*! The skin on his lower legs was so dry that just removing his sock loosened enough scale to be clearly visible in the light of the examining room.

The next exchange confirmed the *cause* of Sid's dry skin. "Sid, tell me, what soap do you use?" He named one of the most popular anti-bacterial "deodorant" soaps on the market, which is advertised on virtually every prime-time TV show. And as most dermatologists are learning, these soaps are some of the most drying influences on human skin ever developed.

In fact, I once treated a little child with severe eczema who was so dry that when you brushed a finger over his skin in good light, you could see the scales fall like snow from his scratched and bleeding little arm. I asked the mother what she had been doing for the dryness, and she

---

Youth Alert!

With increasing age, the moisture content of the dead layer of our skin drops precipitously to near zero. No wonder we're dry in the winter!

---

told me she had been using this same soap *three times daily*—and on the advice of her pediatrician, yet!

A *Little Bathing Goes a Long Way*

So I asked Sid the only logical question. "How *often* are you bathing, Sid, and do you take baths or showers?"

"Aw, c'mon, doc, I bathe every day, and sometimes twice a day—doesn't everybody? I just *love* those hot showers! Why, aren't I supposed to bathe every day? Whaddaya want me to do, stink?"

Hardly. We often tell patients an anecdote about the cavemen. Cavemen didn't suffer from dry, itchy skin. They bathed only once a week, whether they needed it or not! Although I'll admit that that schedule of baths would be prohibitive for most of us who have to work and interact socially every day, it's most important to realize that we *may* be able to skip a bath or two every day or so. Sponge baths can supplement showers. This is especially important if your skin itches and scales. In the following sections, I'll present a nine-point plan for staying completely free of dry skin each and every winter.

My Foolproof Anti–Dry Skin Program

Here's my plan:

1. *Use a humidifier, or another alternative.* One of the chief reasons we have dry skin is the low humidity in the air, which allows our own skin water to evaporate. The solution to this is to try to increase the humidity in the areas where we spend the majority of our time, like bedroom and office. To do this at home, the most efficient way is to buy a whole-house humidification system, which is incredibly effective and healthy for the wintertime. Keep the humidity at about 30%-40% and you'll feel a lot warmer

and moister all winter. You can get one of these systems for a couple of hundred dollars—a wonderful investment.

If you can't afford this, some patients have a good deal of success with small humidifiers put in the rooms at home where they spend the most time. Lacking that, even putting out large pans of water can improve the situation. If you have radiators, put the pans on them so that evaporation is greater. Keep a pan of water boiling on the stove (careful of the children with both of these ideas!). I've even had some patients with small apartments tell me they did very well by leaving a half inch of fresh water in the bathtub! Try it! What have you got to lose except the flakes on your itchy skin?

2. *Cut down on the numbers of baths you take.* There's nothing that makes the problem of dry skin worse than too-frequent bathing. And there's almost no task harder for the dermatologist who understands the mechanisms of dry skin than convincing patients this is important. To do so, we have to fight the constant bombardment of modern cosmetic advertising, which preaches that we will offend if we don't scrub ourselves with wire brushes and the most fragrant anti-bacterial soaps we can possibly find each night.

3. *Take baths instead of showers—and the cooler the better*! The bath is really an honorable institution—people have been getting along with it for a thousand years! But for some reason, except for "recreational use," we've almost given up on the bath. People feel they are not really clean when they take a bath. They seldom, however, consider the downside to taking showers. Think of it for a minute. A shower is like taking a million infinitely small baths—and each and every one of them washes off our natural moisture that we had taken many hours to develop! In a real sense, we can virtually *wash* ourselves into a flaky oblivion with enough showers.

Baths are a different story altogether. A bath does not wash off *all* the natural skin oil. And almost nobody takes a bath as hot as he takes showers! When you think about it, keeping the temperature of a bath up to that near-scalding heat we commonly use for our showers is really difficult.

What's the evidence that showers are terrifically more drying than baths? The worst and most persistent cases of dry skin we see are on the central upper back of tall, white males. This spot has been described by some as the "itchy spot that nobody can reach." The fact is that it's a simple human tendency to stand with one's back toward the shower, with the hot water constantly beating down on the central upper back skin. This practice is torture for the upper back skin, which, day after day, gets all its precious protective oil washed right off. Then the upper dead layer of the skin dries out so that the water content of that layer is almost *zero*! And unless that softening oil is replaced by a moisturizer after the bath, the upper back will become flaky and itchy within minutes, and remain so for hours or even days.

4. *Use the mildest soap you can get your hands on.* There are very few options here. Soap is by definition irritating, because the one thing it's built to do best is what your skin does not need: removing oil! Does removing oil and, therefore, drying out the skin need to be an integral part of cleansing? Absolutely not! It's only logical to try to use a milder cleansing system that actually *replaces* some of the oil that is removed. Most of the soaps we use are so drying that sometimes dermatologists think they were *designed* to hurt the skin. Sure, I know that those sweet-smelling anti-bacterial soaps are popular because of the deodorant claims made about them, but they are the worst and most drying soaps known. And in fact, many of them contain antibiotics to help them fight the bacteria that cause odor—antibiotics which, in the sunlight, can cause an intense rash, called photodermatitis. So these soaps are the ones to definitely *avoid* at all costs.

What's the mildest soap, then? While *no* soap is *good* for your skin, despite what the commercials say, it *is* possible to cleanse the skin and replace some of the oil at the same time. Soaps that are supergentle and do this are Dove, Basis, Neutrogena Dry Skin Formula, and Lowila. And of all these, the ones I've found to be the most useful in my patients is Dove. In two separate tests it's been found to be the mildest soap in human history. And clinical dermatologists will vouch for this anytime. Almost no other soap has the ability to restore moisture to the skin like Dove. I've been using it in my patients for 14 years, and frankly, there's just nothing like it!

Problems with Dove? Very, very few, but the most frequent complaint is the fragrance of the soap. Many people reject it out of hand because of its perfumey smell, and I have almost no success whatsoever in getting men to use it. Happily, the Lever Brothers Company has responded to my requests to produce Dove without fragrance. The new bars were test-released to dermatologists at the December 1988 meeting of the American Academy of Dermatology, and will be on the shelves coincident with the publication of this book. What a responsive company! Thanks, Lever Brothers!

The other soaps I've mentioned are for those folks who have problems with Dove. Among the other soaps, Lowila seems to be the patient's choice for mildness, and Basis and Neutrogena come next.

5. *Consider using a soapless cleanser as a substitute for washing with soap and water.* What about people who just can't tolerate soap? For them, I advise soapless, oil-free skin cleansers like Cetaphil or SFC (which stands for "soap-free cleanser"). I've discussed them in Chapter 4, and Cetaphil is covered extensively in my previous book, *Skin Secrets*. This is an exceedingly gentle and effective way to cleanse the skin without drying it out too much.

Basically, the method consists in rubbing on a light coating of the lotion, nearly lathering it up, and then wiping it off with a tissue. This leaves the skin moist and supple, and causes no excess dryness. It's a way to cleanse and moisturize at the same time.

6. *Use a bath oil, but apply it correctly*. Note, I said "apply," not "pour into bath water," or "pour onto washcloth," as so many of the label directions for these products read. If you put a bath oil into the water of your bath, you lose almost all its effect. Most of it goes right down the drain when you pull the plug. But you *can* get every ounce of good out of your bath oil if you apply it to your wet skin after the bath. Make sure you step *outside* of the bathtub before doing this, because oil on the slippery porcelain can lead to slipping and falling.

7. *Use the right moisturizer*. One would think that with all the products for softening and moisturizing the skin on the market, it would be easy to to stay soft and supple. But, in fact, there are *so* many products that there's no way to pick one intelligently. How do you really find the best one? Ask your dermatologist. Take this book along to his office next time you go, and ask him what he thinks of my recommendations.

I'll say unequivocally that the best moisturizer I've ever seen is Complex-15. This is the same lotion I have used for years to clear up severe eczema in children, even *without* adding cortisone to the mixture. I've been using this product personally and in my patients for years, with more success than any other one on the market. Of course, Complex-15 is not a *cure* or a panacea for dry skin. We all get drier as we age. But it *is* a modern miracle of chemistry that can make dry, harsh, itchy, scaly skin livably comfortable almost any time of the year.

8. *Use protection from the cold at every opportunity*. Protecting skin from the ravages of wind and cold is most difficult, but it *can* be done. To do this best, I advise the double-layer application technique, in which you apply two thin layers of moisturizer, rather than one heavy one. In my patients this has been a vast help in getting the moisturizer to work longer. For runners who are battering

their skins in the cold during all hours of the day, I often advise the two layers of moisturizer, a heavy layer of Vaseline, and even a soft cotton face mask. Don't forget to wear a sunscreen even on winter days to prevent further radiaging damage.

9. *See your dermatologist if the above measures fail in two weeks to solve your dry skin problem.* Realize that if your case of dry skin doesn't appear to be healing in a week or two, you may, in fact, have something *else*, and that's the main reason for getting checked. And if it *is* just a severe case of dry skin, then the dermatologist can do a hundred things with as many medicines to get you well and keep you well.

If all else fails, take this book in to the dermatologist and ask him if he'd consider making you up a prescription for some of the best lotion for treating the most severe cases of dry skin I've ever seen. I call it K.I.L., which stands for Kenalog in (Complex-15) Lotion. Used mainly on the legs and arms, this wonderful stuff is known as the "fire extinguisher" in my office, because of its effectiveness in quelling the itch of dry skin and eczema. It is *not* to be applied to the face, neck, or groin, nor is it for casual use in someone with just a mild case of "winter itch." But for those with severe dry dermatitis, it cannot be beaten. If your dermatologist desires a good formula for mixing up this lotion, have him send me a SASE at the address at the front of this book. Then you can take his prescription to the pharmacist who will mix the lotion for you.

Three Generations of Moisturizers

What makes Complex-15 so effective? It belongs to what I call the third generation of moisturizers. The first generation was the simple bath oils that women have used for thousands of years. These were simply splashed on after the bath, and for a few hours would do a fairly good

<hr>

Youth Alert!

*Only the skin's oil layer prevents dry, itchy skin.
Wash it off without replacing it, and in no time your
skin will feel like cinders!*

<hr>

job of keeping the skin moist. But oils rub off easily, so a new idea was needed.

The second generation of moisturizers came along in the 1940s, with the invention of oil-in-water emulsions. These were lotions in which the oils were contained in small enough drops to stay in solution, not separating back into layers of water and oil. The water tended to moisturize the skin, and the oil acted as a sealant, temporarily preventing the evaporation of water from the skin's dead layer.

A short explanation of that oil layer is in order here. Imagine that you were going away on vacation, and wanted to perform a little "water test." You fill two pie pans half full with water; over one, you place a layer of plastic food wrap. You then leave on your 10-day vacation, and when you get back, you check to see if there is any water left in the pie pans. Do I need to ask you which one would have the water in it? That same function of protection from water evaporation is performed by the oil layer on your skin. Ordinarily, your own sebum from your oil glands would do this job, just as it did for those cavemen we talked about earlier. But sebum, as Dr. Kligman says, "is a really lousy moisturizer. It's Nature's mistake," because of the poor job it does for the skin. Luckily, the newer moisturizers are superior in all respects.

And that brings us to a discussion of the *third-generation moisturizers*, those containing phospholipids, like Complex-15. Phospholipids are long-chained compounds that have two very different molecular ends. One end has a phosphorous group, which is highly attracted to water.

The other end is an oil-loving substance that hangs on tightly to the skin. What a perfect combination! One end grabs the skin itself, and the other end holds onto, or "complexes," 15 molecules of water (hence the name) for every molecule of the active phospholipid. In this way, as tests in the frigid cold of the Philadelphia winter and the dry heat of the Arizona desert have shown, the skin will stay moisturized, even up to *10 days* after using it! Not bad for a chemical harvested from soybeans. It's this soybean derivative that makes Complex-15 one of the most effective moisturizers in history.

Don't get me wrong—there are many good moisturizers. Among the best, some of which were also recommended in Chapter 4, are Moisturel, Purpose, Eucerin, Lubriderm, and Neutrogena. If you have really bad dry skin, especially on the thick areas, like the heels, feet, hands, and arms, you may need the extra potency of the only *prescription* moisturizer, Lac-Hydrin. This is a 12% lactic acid lotion. Lactic acid is a "fruit acid," or alpha-hydroxy acid. These acids (found in fruit) greatly soften the keratin protein layer of the skin's dead layer, causing it to feel much softer and smoother the longer the medicine is used. There is even one nonprescription lotion, Lacticare, which, like Lac-Hydrin, has lactic acid, but in a much lower concentration. If you have very *severe* dry skin, you should give these two a try, but remember that Lac-Hydrin is a prescription item for which you'll have to see the doctor, Lacticare has somewhat less of the active acid ingredient, so it may be purchased over the counter at the drugstore. The reason Lac-Hydrin is a prescription-only product is that some people get significant stinging from it, so it was decided to keep it under the prescription drug law.

More Moisturizer Facts

Here are four more facts you should know about lotions and moisturizers.

======= *Youth Alert!* =======

Never use any skin product containing vitamin E or aloe. To do so is to risk a severe skin allergy.

1. *It's not necessary to pay $60 an ounce for a good moisturizer.* Often (and paradoxically), the more expensive lotions can be frankly damaging to skin because of the many chemicals added to preserve the lotion, which have to be sorted out should an allergic reaction occur. We see examples of this almost daily in the office, especially with lotions that contain vitamin E and aloe—both pretty potent causes of skin allergy, in my experience. The take-home message? Never apply either of these substances to your skin.

Also, and you just wouldn't think that this would happen in this country, I have (on occasion) requested from the manufacturer the exact ingredients for a compound or lotion or fragrance for patch testing on an allergic patient, and I've been *denied*! The company would state that to reveal the ingredient would violate its rules on disclosing proprietary information. As you can understand, that leaves the dermatologist in the difficult position of not being able to tell the patient exactly what the cause of his rash is. Thankfully, the Cosmetic, Fragrance, and Toiletries Association is now regularly coming to the aid of the dermatologist to act as a resource for the exact information needed about certain compounds so that we may test accurately for allergy to each ingredient.

A short aside here on the best companies that produce the best of the moisturizers. These companies, like the Schering Company that makes Complex-15, and the Westwood Company that makes Moisturel and Lac-Hydrin, and the very thorough Neutrogena and Allercreme companies, as well as a few of the more popular brands, like Clinique and Elizabeth Arden products, really *do* help us

========= *Youth Alert!* =========

If you find a really good lotion for any one part of the body, it should be usable on any other part of the body, including the face.

find non–allergy-causing ingredients in their over-the-counter lotions, moisturizers, and cosmetics.

2. *Any good moisturizer should be usable anywhere on the body*—heels as well as eyelids (the limited exception to this is Lac-Hydrin, which, as a potent prescription moisturizer, may cause some stinging if used in softer areas of the body). You don't need special lotions for different areas. And the fact of the matter is, most lotions that designate a part of the body as their "target area" really can be used almost anywhere. But the companies use the area designations to increase revenue, since they'd rather sell a person two or three moisturizers (face and body, for instance) than one.

3. *Collagen in a lotion is no help whatsoever.* When injectable collagen came on the market for correction of wrinkles in the superficial skin, cosmetic companies got the cynical idea that they could make the public believe putting collagen into a lotion would increase its effectiveness. They now peddle *millions* of dollars' worth of lotions with collagen in them every year, doing no more for the patient than increasing the cost. Collagen, as noted in Chapters 3 and 9, is the leathery substance of the skin. There's absolutely no way at all to get it *into* the skin by applying it! The companies claim that its presence in lotions increases their ability to hang onto moisture on the patient's skin, but in reality all they do is make a slurry mess on the *surface* of the skin, not *within* it.

The same goes for all the other useless ingredients in lotions, like elastin, pulverized placenta parts, and amniotic fluid, junk that's put into them to raise the price. It's disgusting to read the lists of ingredients on some of these products! Sometimes I'm amazed that someone hasn't determined some magical effect of pasteurized cow pies in cosmetics! Maybe I shouldn't say that—we'll probably find it on the market next week!

4. *Aloe (the "burn plant") has never been seen to do anything favorable for human skin.* In fact, I often see topical contact allergies to aloe. When this happens, the skin swells and blisters, just like a severe case of poison ivy—it's not a pretty sight, especially on the face.

Remember that air conditioning turns "winter itch" into "all-year itch!" Really try using the advice in my nine-point program. You'll love your soft, supple skin again!

15

The Real Fountain

*Inactivity in the aging population is lethal
business.*
—Albert M. Kligman, MD

Our definition of body aging, not just skin aging, has begun
to change over the last few years. Dr. Lynne Smith, noted
aging researcher, defines it this way: Aging is the gradual
changes in the structure of an organism that occur with
the passage of time, that do not result from disease.
Recently, however, I think the view that aging may be
"normal" has changed. Many of us consider aging to be a
disease in the true sense of the word, in that it does indeed
cause us "*dis*-ease!" This view was confirmed in the spring
of 1988, at a conference of the world's top aging experts
that altered my view of aging forever.

The Biology of Human Skin Aging (hereafter called the
SAG) conference was one of the most exciting dermatological conferences I've ever attended. From the title alone,
many dermatologists decided not to attend, thinking, as
many practicing dermatologists seem to do, that it would
be another meeting of academic minds, spewing forth facts
by the thousands, none of which would be of *practical* use.
But if a doctor were to have carefully read the list of fac-
ulty members and subjects addressed at that meeting, he
would have changed his mind.

This meeting, sponsored by the Jefferson Medical College (one of the world's true pioneers in medical educa-

=== *Youth Alert!* ===

Certainly intrinsic aging (non-radiaging) will always progress, but researchers are beginning to think of the changes that accompany natural aging as true diseases, in that they cause tremendous discomfort in our later years.

tion), gathered the world's most brilliant skin aging researchers, like the now famous Dr. Albert Kligman (discoverer of Retin-A) from the Department of Dermatology at the University of Pennsylvania, who are active, practicing physicians intent on providing useful material for those of us who are, day to day, fighting off the onslaughts of chronic radiaging. And many of the facts revealed at the conference were entirely new to me (a fact that emphasizes how vital it is for private practitioners to get out of their offices and *go* to such conferences to keep up with all the latest developments).

Many of the skin-related facts from that conference have already been stated in previous chapters of this book, but in this chapter I'll tell you about some of the exciting work going on to elucidate the very molecular bases for aging, and maybe, just maybe to slow the body's entire aging process, a goal never previously thought attainable.

Life Span vs. Life Expectancy

Is there a difference between life span and what we most often refer to as life expectancy? There surely is, and the difference is crucial. *Life expectancy* is what we think of when we think of life insurance companies, and the news reports we hear every year that say it's increasing steadily. It's how long the average American can really expect to live. This even varies with sex of the person in question. But *life span* is like an apparent "lid" on human life poten-

Youth Alert!

We truly are on the verge of actually extending our life span, not only by the normal measures we already know about but through some truly astounding discoveries related to the very biochemistry of aging itself!

tial—the number of years beyond which human beings just do not live. And that's the number that's being most closely examined in this chapter.

Of course, there are hundreds of reasons that chemicals, cells, tissues, and people age, and I'm not trying to cover all those theories in this book, but I thought it helpful to point you in the direction of current research, especially as it relates to the questions of therapy that can increase our life span.

I asked a friend and gerontologist (aging specialist) one day what the practical limits of human life were.

"Jerry," I asked him, staring at his own graying temples, "just how long can we make it?"

At first he hedged, because of recent medical advances, transplants, artificial organs, and so on. But after a lot of thought he said, "Joe, I've thought about this for a long time, and I figure we've got about a hundred years' life in us, max. Sure, you hear an occasional story about the 105-year-old, or very rarely, 107 or 115, but for the most part," he said almost apologetically, "we seem to just run out of steam at about a hundred—assuming, that is, that we can hold out *that* long."

Youth Alert!

Many aging specialists feel there is a practical limit to the human lifespan: about 115 years.

"But what about those folks in the Soviet Union who are supposed to be 140 or so, and the Asian mountain peoples who are reported to reach that age?"

"No proof, Joe, no proof. No one has *ever* been able to dredge up any adequate documentation that anyone's ever lived that long!"

I was already a little dismayed, when he said, "But who really cares, Joe? How many of us are really in good enough *shape* to want to live that long in these bodies, anyway?"

I kept thinking of the comment my dive buddy made about how using Retin-A to correct the ravages of radiaging was like putting a 40-year paint job on a 4-year car.

In so many ways, *he was right*, I thought later. If you'll just look around you and see how *some* people age, it is indeed discouraging. I'm reminded, as I write this, of the many times in my office practice I've tried to be encouraging to a very old person, by telling him to see me again in five or six years. Hundreds of times I've heard comments like, "Oh no you won't. Take a good look at me, doc! In this conditon, I wouldn't even *want* to be around that long!" Others, though, have been more positive, seemingly because they are actually *aging better*—more *successfully*, I'd say! What's the difference in the two groups? Is it all genetic? What's the chemistry behind the aging of the human *body* as well as the skin?

And why does a human live 100 years, yet a turtle can live 200? On the other hand, why do dogs die at 10 to 20 years, and chimps die at 45 years? Or more interesting, why do big dogs tend to die earlier than small dogs? Yet the chimp ages qualitatively the same (in exactly the same *way*) as does a human, with many of the same biological problems that occur with aging!

These differences are some of the most confounding of all biologic controversies, and it's taken a long time to get any sort of a handle on them.

Richard G. Cutler, PhD, a researcher from the National Institute on Aging who spoke at the SAG conference, puts it this way: Aging is a problem (certainly a normal one,

```
════════ Youth Alert! ════════

  Aging may be the result of genes, chemicals, envi-
  ronment, diet, and immunity—and, to some extent,
  is related to all these factors. Understandably, pin-
  pointing the exact causes may take many more years.
  A useful book about aging and immunity is Dr.
  Arnold Fox's Immune for Life (Prima, 1989).
```

but still a problem, to be sure) that occurs in every species. The real trick is to figure out why different species age at different rates, and use that knowledge to help us live longer, healthier, more productive lives.

The Best of the Aging Theories

Although there are several major theories on aging and why it occurs, a few stand out as the most plausible. One is that our *immune systems* fail slowly and gradually with the passing of the years. This permits diseases and cancers to strike us much more easily with time. An interesting fact seems to bear this out, at least in part: We all produce tens, if not hundreds, of "cancers" (abnormally proliferating cells) over our lifetimes, each of which could result in our death. It's our finely tuned immune systems that methodically wipe out these cancers and permit us to survive. When operating correctly, this defender of our cells and chemicals against disease is phenomenally powerful. But with age it does decrease in its ability to defend the body—just like an aging battalion of soldiers.

Another theory says the genetic material of the cells and the chemicals that keep those genes operating efficiently just wear out with age. If true, this would result in the aging cells' gradually decreasing in their normal functions, until life could no longer be supported.

<hr>

===== *Youth Alert!* =====

*Even some of the body's normal reactions cause
"loose cannons" which are constantly damaging our
body's chemistry!*

<hr>

Oxyradicals: Life's Invisible Thugs

Yet another major theory involves a crucial class of compounds called *oxyradicals*, extremely reactive molecules produced during the metabolism of oxygen. They are defined as any molecule with an "unpaired electron." Let me explain this in a little more detail. If you've forgotten your high school chemistry, all molecules are composed of protons and neutrons in the nucleus, and electrons circling around the nucleus like tiny planets. In order for two molecules to "react," or bind together ("bond"), one molecule combines a free electron with a free electron from another molecule, forming a pair of electrons—a very stable arrangement in nature.

Some reactions in the body's energy/respiration system, however, produce oxygen molecules with a free, *unpaired* electron—a highly unstable arrangement. Like the neighborhood bully who'd attack anyone, just for a fight, this high-energy atom is able to temporarily bond with almost every one of the body's vital chemicals, without being destroyed itself.

So oxyradicals, then, are the body's dangerous natural pollutants—*internal* pollutants that are in you and me right this very minute, reacting chemically with almost every one of the body's precious life-sustaining chemicals. They are like indiscriminate robbers who race down our bodies' streets and throw acid on everyone they see, ruining them for life. You can't feel them, and you can't see them, but they're there.

And aging *differences*, it seems, may be related to how effectively we develop our chemical police forces to deal with these bandits. Some species, like the turtles, appear to have superb gendarmes patrolling the streets to quench, soak up, or capture these invasive and destructive oxyradicals, but those that do not develop such mechanisms are doomed to die earlier—sometimes *much* earlier, like the chimp, who zips through all the changes of human aging twice as fast as we do.

Where do these abominable chemical criminals come from? Is it possible to stop them at their point of origin? Sadly enough, it is not (as yet) possible to limit the production of these marauders, because they are the natural products of our oxygen metabolism—that is, they come from entirely normal chemical reactions transpiring in our bodies 24 hours of every day. These are the very reactions that define life—and how ironic that the very product of life is death; that we begin aging at the moment of fertilization, and from that instant our existence is measured in and by the chemicals we produce.

Life spans of cells, then, which Dr. Cutler aptly calls "Life Span Energy Potential," differ in different species by how well each species develops a police force to fight these oxyradicals. If the fight is *not* very effective, life span is much shorter, as in the lowly tree shrew who lives only eight years. Species that vigorously combat oxyradicals, like the turtles we mentioned, live tremendously longer lives.

Why do these chemicals make such a difference? Because they attack the genetic material of the cells—the very stuff of life, which controls exactly how long each cell will be viable.

So in a definite sense, says Dr. Cutler, aging depends on adequate defenses against oxyradicals. Yet oxyradicals are products of perfectly normal (and unchangeable) reactions in the body. How does the body accomplish this defense?

Again, chemicals come into play to "squelch" these criminals. Four such chemicals are vitamins E, A, and C, and beta-carotene. These chemicals, at least in part, are some of the main biologic defenses against oxyradicals.

Are Vitamins the Answer?

Once you've heard this, a few questions should immediately pop into your mind. We certainly have limitless sources of these vitamins. Would it not be logical to take additional vitamins A, C, E, and beta-carotene? Nobody knows for sure, but it *appears* that some extension of the limits of life might result from doing this.

I'm quick to add, however, that the experts suggest that taking extra vitamins of this type may have what the scientists call a "negative feedback" effect. That means if you *provide* additional amounts of these vitamins, the body may just decrease its *own* output of the protective molecules, so the net effect on oxyradicals may be essentially unchanged. And even more important, some of the fat-soluble vitamins (vitamins D, E, A, K) are actually *toxic* in high doses! Therefore, *no one should increase their own intake of these specific vitamins without the specific advice of his doctor*. Vitamin A, especially, has some alarming side effects, everything from mild lip chapping to elevation of the fats in the blood, fetal malformations, severe headaches, and even bone pain. So don't load up on vitamin supplements. Remember the saying that "the person who treats himself has a fool for a patient!"

We Should All Be "SOD-Busters"

What we really need more of is the second class of the body's controllers of oxyradicals, the enzymes called superoxide dismutase (SOD) and catalase, which are produced in varying amounts by each of the body's cells. These

Youth Alert!

Do not *adjust your intake of vitamins on the basis of what you'll read here. We have no long-term studies of such a plan in humans. I mention the beneficial effect of such chemicals simply so you'll be aware of recent research, not so you'll load up on vitamins without your doctor's advice.*

enzymes are present in much greater quantities in relatively long-living species. But scientists have not as yet devised any ways to produce more SOD or catalase in our systems. Health food stores have been known to sell SOD tablets, but there is no proof that *any* of it gets into the system or into the cells where the oxyradicals are found.

The other factor that controls longevity is the efficient repair of damaged DNA, that stuff of life which controls the replication of all our bodies' cells. Perhaps those who live longer not only have more SOD but carve out damaged sections of DNA more efficiently, allowing the normal chemical structures to be rebuilt. We know that some diseases exist, like xeroderma pigmentosum, in which amounts of DNA-repairing enzymes are notoriously low, resulting in skin disasters (early aging: multiple deadly skin cancers starting very early in life). Such diseases pave the way for a chemical model of aging, in which failure to repair damage, and not just creation of damage, is to blame.

Sugar: Another of Our Slow Executioners

Another series of fascinating observations was made at the SAG conference by Dr. Anthony Cerami, concerning the havoc glucose causes in the aging onslaught. Glucose is the sugar of which we all need a constant and stable

======= *Youth Alert!* =======

Pigments (or comparable cross-links of chemicals)
formed by the reaction of glucose with other body
molecules may be some of the chief chemicals
responsible for old age.

supply minute to minute in all our body fluids and tissues.
Nobody ever believed it could be the culprit in *any* disease, except diabetes, and even there, glucose long seemed
only a victim of upset insulin production and release.
However, those theories as to the importance of that sugar
have radically changed our thinking of its role, at least in
Dr. Cerami's experiments.

To use Dr. Cerami's example, think of what happens
when you cook a turkey in the oven. The pale meat of the
bird warms gradually, and finally browns with the intense
heat of the oven. That's what we want, naturally, and that's
what makes the turkey appetizing. In other words, it's a
normal chemical reaction of cooking (one that does not
occur very readily, by the way, in microwave cooking, currently the subject of much intense work to *make* the
browning occur!). The actual brownness is caused by pigments formed when sugars in the turkey combine with
other compounds (protein, fats, DNA, and others). This
reaction is called *glycosolation*. In the case of cooking, the
glycosolation happens due to heat, while in many normal
circumstances in the body, glycosolation occurs with the
help of enzymes that speed the reaction along in a harm-
less way.

Cerami noted, however, that some of the unwanted glucose pigments occur without enzymes *or* heat in normal
people, and he showed some striking examples of this
happening.

One of his slides showed a sample of serum from the
blood of a normal youth. It was crystal clear. The same

======= *Youth Alert!* =======

> *Diabetics undergo many apparent age-related*
> *changes much sooner than the "normal" population.*
> *This may be related to the generally higher levels of*
> *glucose present in their bodies, and the reaction of*
> *that glucose with many body proteins necessary to*
> *keep us young.*

sample from an elderly patient showed a clear-cut tan color, a pigment (which many, in fact, call "age pigment") remaining in the normally clear serum. It was proof of a special nonenzymatic type of glycosolation, which occurs in all of us with time, even without heat or enzymes to activate the reaction.

Diabetics Show Accelerated Aging

Diabetics show many of the changes of aging faster than the rest of the population. And as a corollary to that statement, the worse the control of the blood sugar in a diabetic, the earlier and more severe are these changes. The second fact hit those of us at the SAG conference like a load of bricks: The serum from a young, badly controlled diabetic tested similarly showed a deep tan, almost *brown* coloration, indicating vast amounts of the combined glucose-protein pigments had already accumulated.

It's not that the body has absolutely no defense against these pigments—that is not true. "Scavenger cells," called macrophages, normally digest small amounts of the pigments as they are produced, but even these efficient little scavengers can't keep up with the full load of pigments produced with age. So they accumulate ever so slowly in the normal person, and much more quickly in the diabetic.

The significance is this: Think of how many conditions are commonly associated with aging—atherosclerosis and

---

Youth Alert!

Your proteins actually get "stiffer" with age, due to cross-linking with sugar molecules!

---

arteriosclerosis, certainly, are the first two to come to mind, but others are also common. Think of how an old person walks, with rigid joints and stiffening tissues around them. Isn't that a strikingly consistent sign of aging? Couldn't that be accounted for, at least in part, by the cross-linking of these glucose-protein pigments? It certainly could! It would be like pouring Super Glue on a rope. The analogy holds with many diseases of aging, as you might imagine. And other conditions immediately jump to mind, such as cataracts, osteoporosis, hypertension, malignancies, autoimmune diseases, and many other age-associated conditions, in which the joining of glucose with DNA, protein, and other vital body substances occurs.

Now consider this: All of the above problems occur at *much earlier* ages in many diabetics! That suspicion, now being proved by researchers like Dr. Cerami, has been the very principle of treatment for diabetics under strict management and control of blood sugar in such institutions as the Joslin Clinic. This center of excellence in diabetic management espouses exacting control of blood sugar in order to try to prevent the horrendous and insidious complications of that disease from setting in.

Youth Alert!

For diabetics, of course, the tighter the rein kept on the blood sugar level the better. And for the rest of us, compounds are being found that can block the negative effect of blood sugar.

Youth Alert!

Glucose, by reacting insidiously with DNA in our bodies, may be breaking that substance into fragments, thus causing mutations and probably cancers and many other problems.

A little side note about a diabetes test: One test for the accuracy of a diabetic's long-term control looks at the number of glucose-hemoglobin molecules that are carried in the red blood cells. This test actually measures glucose combined nonenzymatically with the chief blood compound, hemoglobin, which forms, similar to the food pigments we've mentioned, a brownish coloration. This measures how well a person's blood sugar has been under control for the whole previous month.

Proof that this reaction occurs in all bodies can be seen in the changing color of cartilage. A pure whitish color in youth, it turns a yellowish-brown with age. This color, too, is a function of chemical reactions of glucose with protein. These multiple examples of glucose combining with our proteins indicate a reaction that occurs in many different tissues. The real problem, caused by the stiffness in tissues produced by this cross-linking, is that DNA can be broken or altered. As a result, DNA's repairability decreases, causing all sorts of mutations and internal disasters that can lead to cancers and other complications. The upshot of all this is that glucose is actually responsible for some *mutations* in the human body.

Treating the "Glucose Connection"

We know that these deadly reactions between glucose and other substances occur, but what can you do about it? You can't get rid of glucose; that's what keeps us all alive. But

Youth Alert!

Will science fiction in aging become science fact? I believe it will, and that much of our current research into the causes of aging will produce real advances that will help us all live longer and healthier lives.

maybe scientists and biochemists can help us by designing drugs that will block all the sites of attachment of glucose to major substances, and therefore extend life. One such drug now under investigation, called *aminoguanidine*, binds to the site to which glucose is attracted, and prevents glucose from attaching onto other chemicals vital to normal health.

Aminoguanidine is now in animal testing to determine its toxicity, and may, in one form or another, turn out to be a medicine of choice for aging related to nonenzymatic combination of sugars with proteins. But don't hold your breath! Studies will take many years to complete. It's good to know, though, that science is on the road to a major breakthrough.

Aging and Exercise

What about the role of exercise in age prevention? We already know by some of the brilliant work of Dr. Gary Grove, director of the Skin Study Center in Springfield, Pennsylvania, that activity and movement during all phases of our lives play some role in retarding skin aging. He has proven this unequivocally with an instrument he calls the "twistometer," which grasps the skin on the back of the hands or arms and twists it a fraction of a turn, measuring in the process the force exerted by the skin to return to its original shape. This tensile strength has an assigned number value, being higher in younger skin and lower in older skin. He has found that the skin maintains much more of its youthful tightness in those who stay active and mobile as they age! In other words, the "pinch test" that we discussed earlier in this book actually shows a younger, more elastic result in those who maintain active lifestyles. That's good news, and partially explains why we occasionally see a news report of a pretty darned young-looking 90-year-old setting some running record for his or her age group!

Aging and Eating

While some experiments in lower animals do show life extension on various diets fortified with some of the vitamins and chemicals we've discussed, the only constantly effective way to increase the longevity of those animals was to decrease their caloric intake. It's as if a minor restriction on the diets, so that the animals were never allowed to eat just as much as they would have liked, actually was responsible for the increased lengths of the lives of these animals.

Research may indicate in future years that a form of mild chronic restriction of food, a very mild "starvation," if you will, may help us humans too. We will just have to wait and see. But it's true that this seems to work in many animal systems, and in the meantime, most Americans could benefit from a little food restriction. Perhaps a fortified, slightly restricted diet will be the answer to adding some years to our lives. All I hope is that someone will make dieting a whole lot easier!

There are many and varied reasons why people age, and we don't yet know how to carve out all the keys to extending life—or in fact whether we *want* to. Are Retin-A, vitamins A, C, E, beta-carotene, SOD, catalase, aminoguanidine, and dietary restriction the real "stuff" of life extension? Only time and much more research will tell.

In the meantime, what we *can* do is keep our ears to the ground for the sounds of the onrushing waters that proclaim science has discovered the sources of the Fountain of Youth.

16

Youth Begins with Y-O-U

You can't help getting older, but you don't have to get old!
—*George Burns*

When grace is joined with wrinkles, it is adorable. There is an unspeakable dawn in happy old age.
—*Victor Hugo*

George Burns and Victor Hugo, generations apart, were really saying the same thing. We can't halt the passage of time, but we *can* make those passing moments much more enjoyable.

In this book we've discussed the many changes that occur in the skin and in the body during the aging process. I hope you've come to think about aging in much different terms as a result. This book wasn't meant to usher you comfortably into your later years, but to inspire you to try to hold the line—to "rage, rage against the dying of the light." I urge you to fight aging tooth-and-nail every step of the way.

In the final analysis, people look better and younger not only through what they *do* to themselves and for themselves but through how they *feel* about themselves. Many is the time in my office that I've witnessed a depressed patient looking much older than her years. Here's an example of what I mean.

Youth Alert!

For many who notice the first signs of aging, depression and sadness and stress go hand-in-hand with the appearance of the first wrinkles. And often, almost like magic, these very wrinkles clear spectacularly as the stress is resolved.

Giving Yourself a Psychological Face Lift

Louisa came in for me to help her cure some "sores" (as she called them) on her face and the back of the neck. She spoke ever so slowly, and was quite sad-looking and even tearful at times while she tried to explain the reason for her visit.

When I took a closer look at her sores and her intense distress, and asked a few of questions, I found that she and her husband were splitting up after 15 years of marriage. She had been trying to handle this pretty much on her own, and the stress was just too much for her. She had been sad a long time, and it showed painfully in her facial wrinkles and the spots she called "sores"—spots she was making with her own fingernails! Picking at the sores was a way for her to punish herself for what had gone wrong in her life. But with intense psychotherapy over the next few months, she experienced a striking turnabout in her looks, as the divorce was settled amicably. While the sadness over the breakup of her long marriage lingered for many months, she was able to start socializing again, and as I watched, we both started seeing the wrinkles fading from her face as her lesions healed. Under all that stress, worry, and emotion was a very attractive woman!

Why are these changes so evident? It could be said in a single word: *stress*! Can you doubt that theory? Do you

---

Youth Alert!

Living worry-free, with style and élan, will make your later years intensely more pleasant.

---

dispute that much beauty really *does* come from within, and can be virtually destroyed by stress? Think of how much faster those in positions of intense stress appear to age. Think of how badly our presidents seem to age during their short four to eight years in office (Ronald Reagan excepted!). Think of Richard Nixon, entering office almost as a young man, and leaving it in disgrace nearly six years later looking like death warmed over. But then think of how much better he looks now, some 15 years after that troubled time. Admittedly, he's years older now, and has some signs of intrinsic aging, but the effect of time on the healing of his worry signs on his face is clearly evident.

We know from all the discussion in this book about the physiology of aging that (so far) nothing will alter the inexorable progression of the intrinsic changes that occur in all of us. But we should know from personal experience that one of the chief agers of us all is our attitude. Let's put it this way: Physical beauty will not last forever, not with all the Retin-A and plastic surgery in the world. But a woman with style, or élan, what the French call "je ne sais quoi" (that certain something), will have the ability to transcend mere physical prettiness and emerge as a woman of substance, possessing charm and presence and an inner glow. Such a woman will have the ability to transcend a wrinkle or two with youthful spirit and inner beauty. *This* is what I mean by the title of this chapter. I believe that whether or not you start on Retin-A, or get your leg veins injected, or make your hair grow back with minoxidil, or use the best moisturizer that money can buy, you can still *look* and *feel* young by letting that inner glow shine forth. This is not religious or psychological hokum.

===== *Youth Alert!* =====

Try to stay "connected" as you age—connected to
your spouse and friends above all, but also to the
community and your church, if you have one, so that
you have some firm anchors in your life that will
prompt continued interest and enjoyment with each
passing year.

This works! Many is the time I've seen patients with terrible chronic illnesses who adapt, adjust, and go forward
bravely with their lives with attitudes that enliven and
invigorate us all! And if an arthritic, or a cancer patient,
or a severe diabetic can do it, surely we all can do it.

As noted physician and lecturer Arnold Fox, author of
Immune for Life (Prima, 1989), says:

> There is a direct relationship between one's outlook on life
> and aging. Anger, fear, frustration and other stressful
> thoughts prompt the release of high-voltage substances in
> the body that jolt the heart, weaken the immune system,
> and speed the aging process. On the other hand, in my 30-
> plus years as an internist and cardiologist, I have been struck
> by the beneficial effect that joy, serenity, and peace of mind
> have on the body. How does one develop the positive, healthy
> outlook on life that slows the aging process? It begins with
> the understanding that you are the only one thinking in
> your head. You can choose to see your world through eyes
> of joy and serenity. Or you can do the opposite. I have
> observed that those who chose joy tended to live young,
> healthy, and joyful to a very old age.

Your mental outlook and ability to cope with day-to-
day stresses can have an astounding effect on the way you
are perceived. A woman who smiles constantly will always
be perceived to be younger and more beautiful than one
who frowns constantly. Think of your own experience.
Smilers have a special advantage. People don't tend to see
past the smile to the minor faults that may be present.

Youth Alert!

The best "cosmetic" for aging is a bright, interested smile!

Think to yourself how many times a situation like the one that happened to me today happens to you.

As I write this, I'm on a book tour for my first book, *Skin Secrets*, and I'm traveling on jets all over the East and South. Today one of my planes was late, and I was feeling a little irritated. When I inquired about the status of the flight, I was ready to face a stressful moment with appropriate disgust, but instead, I met a young Delta ticket agent whose bright and cheery smile made a rough wait a lot more tolerable.

I'm not talking about the kind of fruity enthusiasm you see in the plasticized chain restaurants, where the service person approaches you with an insincere "Hi there! My name is John, and I'll be your server for today. What may I serve you?" I've often been tempted to say, "Just iced tea with a little sincerity, please!" I'm talking about an expression of interest—the very sign that you're a person with genuine concern.

How often, I'm sad to say, I've seen this superficiality even in physicians. We tend to approach our five-thousandth patient with a gallstone as "the gallbladder in room 5," instead of a *real* person with *real* problems and concerns. Patients are astute at spotting this, and really know when they've connected with a physician who actually cares about them and their problems. You know the feeling yourself. It's the difference between the doctor who sits down with you and listens with concern, and the guy who grudgingly, as my friend and patient Jane says, "answers all your questions as quickly as possible with one hand on the damned doorknob of the examining room!"

===== *Youth Alert!* =====

*No one would ever insist that you "look your age,"
but you shouldn't try to look atypically young,
either. That's just as bad as premature aging!*

So your smile is indeed your best asset. And it may be a real psychological lift too. Imagine trying to really worry about something with a smile on your face. A smile can give a middle-aged person a sense of inner peace, of knowing who she is and finding her way through life and dealing with it.

Do you like being around someone who constantly complains, and never has a fresh smile for *anybody*? Certainly not. Sales experts learned about this long ago. Look, for instance, at the before-and-after ads for beauty products. They almost universally have the "before" person frowning, or neutral, and the "after" subject with a broad smile on her face. Tells you a lot about the importance of a smile, doesn't it?

Aging should be a natural experience, not one that makes people say, "She's sure had a lot of plastic surgery, hasn't she?" Instead, you'd like people to think how fresh you look for whatever age you are. Anyone who insists on trying to look 29 all her life, with or without plastic surgery, can exude the image of an antiquated gargoyle. You cannot hide all the effects of time, even with all the measures discussed in this book, but you *can* make yourself look as good as you can for *any* age.

Consider Posture and Osteoporosis

Smiles are important, certainly, but consider how much better a smile looks on a body in a state of fine repair. Consider posture, for instance. We all know about the

---

Youth Alert!

You do not have to suffer from osteoporosis to any great degree after menopause. What's the answer? Exercise, and combination therapy with hormones like Premarin and Provera!

---

dowager's hump—the curved spine defect that prompted the term "little old lady," because of the overall loss of height it engenders. This is a sign of osteoporosis, the gradual loss of bone substance seen most prominently in elderly women, but beginning as early as the late 40s in some women. Another symptom of osteoporosis is bone fracture. Fully 40% of elderly women have broken a long bone, a pelvis, or a hip by the age of 75! It happens because of the cessation of estrogen function with menopause, which induces bone loss, but the gynecologic experts I've talked to are universally optimistic that almost never needs to happen.

Osteopororis is *not* preventable by simple calcium supplementation. In other words, the bones cannot be maintained just by *taking* more calcium, no matter what the source of the mineral. But prevention *is* possible, however, in the form of estrogen replacement to stop the inexorable reabsorption of the minerals that make your bones so strong.

How does estrogen replacement work to save bone? And doesn't estrogen cause cancers? Estrogen hormone seems to stop reabsorption of bone. It *is* indeed associated with an increased incidence of uterine cancers, but only when taken alone, without the other major female hormone, progesterone. If a woman takes both, in a cyclical manner as prescribed by her gynecologist, there is *no* associated increase in cancer.

The other main preventive is exercise, which stimulates the millions of little cells that lay down bone to continue

<table>
<tr><td>

══ *Youth Alert!* ══

Don't give up your cosmetics as you age. A simple system can be found for just about everybody, so that you can rid yourself of some of the graying of the years!

</td></tr>
</table>

doing so. This is one of the most marvelous ways to develop and keep sturdy bones in your later years. How much exercise is necessary? Again we turn to the experts, who tell us that walking about two miles daily will be almost entirely protective against osteoporosis.

Think of that! By taking medicine and walking a little, you may prevent this hideous and physically troubling complication of aging, osteoporosis and the broken bones and misery that go along with it. In this regard, you should read the best treatise on women and aging I've ever seen, *How a Woman Ages* by Robin Marantz Henig (Ballantine, 1985). It outlines the general maladies that accompany aging, and it lists a plethora of resources for helping the older person find help with various problems.

Assess Your Looks

With the passing of the years, stand back every once in a while, look into a mirror, and just consider your overall looks. Don't accept the gray skin tone that strikes so many aging people. Don't give up your cosmetics, but don't try to apply them like a teenager applies hers, either. You should try for moderation in amount and color, so that the cosmetics just tend to take the edge off the visible grayness in the face. No cosmetic system can make you a teenager again, but cosmetics can help you feel younger, and that's what counts in the final analysis.

Youth Alert!

If you develop or have developed cataracts as you age, I encourage you to have the necessary surgery to remove them. No, I'm not an ophthalmologist, but I've seen the benefits that follow this operation. Admittedly, all our senses seem to dull somewhat with the passing of the years, but we should do everything we can to preserve sight, the most important of them all.

How do you learn what's appropriate and looks good for your age group? Ask a close friend, or try to find a person in a finer department store who has some time to really help you get into the right colors and the right system for you. If your vision is failing at all, you should keep your cosmetic regimen simple, but remember that vision most often fails in the elderly because of cataracts, and they are highly treatable.

Don't settle for losing your vision from cataracts as you age. A patient once told me that her grandfather developed two severe cataracts at age 80, which prevented him from doing what he most liked to do in life, read his Bible. Since he thought he couldn't possibly have many years left, he declined to have the operation to remove them and replace them with implanted lenses. He kept refusing for 10 more years, and then finally acquiesced to his family's suggestion to have this simple procedure done. He read easily with the help of some thin reading glasses for another *15* years, and finally died in his sleep at *105*!

Getting back to the point about cosmetics: You can look a lot better to yourself and your friends if you seek a little help with a simple cosmetic system. I wouldn't want to appear "ageist" in a book aimed at staying young, but I can tell you that in my vast experience with cosmetics in my practice, a slightly older saleswoman will usually be of much greater help to you in finding the correct system.

Youth Alert!

Dermage cosmetics were designed with aging skin in mind. This system contains not only intense moisturizers but sunscreens to prevent further drying and aging from sun exposure.

As always, someone who thoroughly understands a problem from personal experience is much better equipped to deal with it. Try the Clinique and Elizabeth Arden lines. They have really well-trained, helpful people, although the saleswomen for Clinique are rarely out of their 20s. The other cosmetic system that works well for the elderly is the Dermage system, which is available only from your dermatologist. Make sure, if you ask about Dermage, that the person who demonstrates the products gets you the pearl line—it's a lot less drying for older skin (actually, it was *created* for it!).

Hair Color

Nothing cries "Aging!" more loudly than hair color. The hair thins as the years pile on, and to remedy this, you can do exactly the *opposite* of what many women do, which is to color their hair silver or silver-blue. This is the classic tipoff that the person under the coif is over 70! Avoid too light a color! The lighter the color of the hair, the less it can be seen, and the thinner it looks. After all, why do you think women often bleach the dark "moustache" hair on their upper lips? To make it invisible! And the last thing we want is for your *scalp* hair to be less visible!

But it's essential to avoid too dark a color too. Up to a certain color, darkening the hair will make it appear thicker, but everybody realizes that almost *everyone's* hair gets lighter with advancing age. If you go too dark, you'll

┌───┐
│ ══════════ *Youth Alert!* ══════════   │
│   │
│ *Don't be afraid to keep up with your schedule of* │
│ *permanents as the years pass. Age never demands* │
│ *that you abandon your normal hair care. And* │
│ *remember that a little* gentle *"ratting," or backcomb-* │
│ *ing of the hair will often make it appear very much* │
│ *fuller!* │
│   │
└───┘

look awful, and won't be fooling *anybody*. Remember, we want you to look the best for all your ages, instead of the worst for them. Take a lesson from former President Reagan in this regard: Leave a touch of gray at the temples, and don't go too dark with the color correction.

Exercise

A final note about the Y-O-U in YOUTH. There is nothing more important to keeping you younger than continual exercise—some physical activity that you do regularly each day. One of the chief characteristics we attribute to those who have reached "une certaine age," as the French say, is lack of movement. If you have the fortune to maintain your health in even *reasonably* good status, you can engage in some type of exercise program, whether it be walking in a shopping mall or exercycling at home. But remember this: *All exercise programs in the elderly require an exam by your physician, and his approval before beginning.* There

┌───┐
│ ══════════ *Youth Alert!* ══════════   │
│   │
│ *Getting into the habit of even very* mild *exercise as* │
│ *you age will* greatly *help you keep adjusted and in* │
│ *tune with your body. But remember to see the doc-* │
│ *tor before starting any such routine!* │
│   │
└───┘

should never be an exception to this—your own doctor is your very best adviser. But if you *do* have a regular exercise plan, you may be able to look much younger, even if just by the spring in your step and the tightened muscles that keep your skin from sagging. And you'll feel younger than you would have imagined, partly because the circulation can improve so much with continual exercise. In my own office I'll often see, during the same practice day, elderly patients with very, very different lifestyles—some regular exercisers and some not. Those who exercise almost universally have better color, as well as firmer muscles, and a generally better outlook on where they stand in their lives.

As we age, we all want to improve our appearance and well-being. It is my fervent hope that, through the use of this book, you will attain some of the benefits and "Youth Miracles" science and medicine are currently giving us. Remember, the goal of this book is for you to be the least likely in your age group to prompt a discussion of the subject of "aging." Let me know how you're doing. I'd love to hear. Good luck, and good health.

APPENDIX

Other Uses for Retin-A

*In dermatology, if you have had 10 years'
experience, and if you don't know the
diagnosis one foot away in one minute, you
are not going to know it in three hours.*
—Albert M. Kligman, MD

By now I hardly have to tell you what an amazing drug Retin-A is. But you may be surprised to learn that it has been used successfully for many, many diseases besides acne and radiaging. This appendix is designed to tell you about some of those other uses, in the hope that if you have one of the diseases or conditions mentioned here, you'll discuss with a dermatologist their treatment not only with Retin-A, but also with the many other means available.

FDA Approval

Please be aware, as I have said many times in this book, that Retin-A is *not* FDA-approved for these conditions, just as it is *not* FDA-approved for the treatment of radiaging or premalignancies, both of which it helps tremendously. Remember, "FDA-non-approved" does *not* mean *ineffective*. In fact, the reverse is true, largely because the drug companies realize that dermatologists are innovative people and will, by their very natures, investigate the

========= *Youth Alert!* =========

"Middle-age blackheads" are helped by avoidance of sunlight and oils in the workplace. Sulfur soaps, benzoyl peroxide, acne surgery, and most of all, Retin-A have proved most effective in treating this problem.

use of drugs in diseases for which they were never originally intended.

Now, let's talk about some of those conditions in which Retin-A has been tried.

Middle-Age Facial Blackheads

Facial blackheads are often seen in middle and old age, especially on the faces of men who work around cutting oils and other petroleum products. These dark, ugly black dots are usually seen on the upper outer cheeks and temples, and are often accompanied by dozens of blackheads and whiteheads on the eyelids as well. This syndrome, called "cutaneous elastoidosis with cysts and comedones" or "Favre-Racouchot Syndrome," is a solar, environmental, and genetic problem that's incredibly stubborn.

Until Retin-A came on line, all dermatologists could do for this condition was suggest potent sulfur soaps, benzoyl peroxides, and acne surgery. Acne surgery still plays an important part, since in this technique, the dermatologist actually pushes out, or expresses, the oily contents of these jammed-up oil glands.

Thanks to another of Dr. Albert Kligman's studies, it was discovered that application of a solution of Retin-A could erase all the blackheads and whiteheads, and that using the medicine every few days would maintain clear skin in these very susceptible areas. I have used Retin-A and acne surgery, sometimes combined with sulfur soaps,

========== *Youth Alert!* ==========

Non–whitehead-causing moisturizers are critical for use in anyone over 40 who uses Retin-A. See Chapter 4 for recommendations.

in these "senile comedones" many, many times, and I've found Retin-A to be the only topical agent effective for this problem.

Stubborn Whiteheads in Women

Another type of whitehead, found mainly in middle-aged and elderly women, results from chronic use of cold creams and acne-causing cosmetics. These stubborn whiteheads are extremely difficult to get out by just pushing on them with the special instruments used in acne surgery. Their stubbornness and lack of responsiveness to conventional treatments for blackheads shows the astounding ability of the skin to be injured by cosmetics and cleansing creams. Most skin can withstand this type of torture for years before the oil gland openings are irreparably jammed shut by either the substances themselves or the thick oil and sticky cells which they cause the oil glands to produce.

And although it's sometimes difficult to get an elderly woman to use Retin-A because of the slight dryness and irritation it can produce, most women can be started on it intermittently, and the lesions will very slowly open on their own, drain, and fade away. Here, the choice of moisturizer is crucial, not only for the obvious reason that the skin will be dry on Retin-A, but because one must be selected that has absolutely no tendency to induce the skin to form whiteheads and/or blackheads. I have had some significant success with such women patients by asking them to use the mid-strength Retin-A cream (blue and white tube) as their sole night cream, replacing the heavy stuff that probably caused all the whiteheads in the first place.

Beard Bumps (Pseudofolliculitis)

As residents at the Medical College of Georgia, we all took turns rotating out to a stint in the dermatology clinic at Fort Gordon, the local U.S. Army base. Here we were to get our introduction to the varied skin diseases that can occur in a widely dissimilar group of men whose skins were undergoing some truly amazing stresses not ordinarily experienced by our office patients. And believe me, we were introduced, all right!

One of the major problems we had to deal with at the Fort was the problem of "beard bumps" in the black recruits. This horrendous condition is like pustular acne with scarring on the face and occurs because the curly beard hairs of black men often recurve down into the skin, producing intense inflammation. The heat and stresses of physical training, as well as the demand of the training instructors that the recruits shave as closely as possible, made the average black man's face a sort of personal battleground. Luckily for the trainees, we had Retin-A available, which soon eased the infection and inflammation, and as physicians on the base, we regularly put the black recruits "on profile," demanding that they be permitted to grow a quarter-inch beard, a practice which (along with Retin-A usage) was curative in many of the men.

Actinic Keratoses:
Cancers in Our Future

For this problem, two medicines work magnificently together, Retin-A and Efudex. You are certainly acquainted with Retin-A from the first section of this book, but you may not know much about Efudex (5-fluorouracil), a substance that destroys cells which have been made premalignant by chronic sun damage. In cream form, Efudex causes intense redness on the facial skin when it is applied twice a day (the usual dose). The premalignant keratoses, or thickenings on the thin facial skin, grow fiery red as they become irritated by the medicine, but the normal, unaffected skin is completely spared the effects of the medicine. The treatment is continued for three weeks, stopped, and gradually the skin returns to its normal coloration. This works perfectly on the face, removing not only the premalignant keratoses destined to become skin cancers in the future but also the "actinic lentigo," or sun freckles, which cause the brownish, muddied color of so many Caucasian faces.

But the sun, naturally, strikes more than just the face, and that means many other areas also get sun exposure and sunspots. The problem with these areas is that the skin—on the tops of the arms, for instance—is quite thick, and not very amenable to simple Efudex therapy—the medicine just will not get through this thick, damaged skin. This is where Retin-A enters the treatment plan for these special areas of sun damage. Retin-A, applied either before or after the Efudex, causes a greatly intensified penetration of and reaction to Efudex. Used as a double layered treatment, the two drugs will obliterate nearly all premalignant keratoses on the arm and backs of the hands.

In my own practice, this treatment is so effective that I *biopsy* virtually any remaining spot when I see the patient a few months later. I do this, of course, to check for any actual skin cancers that would not normally be eliminated by the Retin-A/Efudex treatment (although some, called superficial basal cell cancers, actually *are* wiped out by it!), but that we might not have been able to see before the treatment.

I've previously mentioned how Retin-A can cause the disorganized, premalignant cells of sun-damaged skin to

---

===== *Youth Alert!* =====

In general, the combination of Retin-A and Efudex is not to be used on the face. That skin is too thin to tolerate it.

---

normalize themselves, but in the case of the Retin-A/Efudex treatment for the backs of hands and arms, it's used more as a penetrating agent, or facilitator of the normal reaction to Efudex. However, without Retin-A added to the regimen, it may take months or *years* to clear up the same keratoses.

Again, be aware that this combination is *not* approved by the FDA for use on actinic keratoses—it's just another of the hundreds of uses for good drugs dermatologists have discovered that *work*, and that we use in patients who need them.

Melasma (Mask of Pregnancy)

Most women have heard of the "mask of pregnancy." These brownish stains on the face can be virtually disfiguring. The condition looks like a superficial stain in the skin (which it is, really), distributed over the upper lip, cheeks, forehead, and even down the arms, occasionally, all the way to the wrists! Because of the darkness of the pigment, some patients have even compared the look of it to the face of a raccoon!

Melasma occurs, for the most part, because of hormonal influences of pregnancy or taking the birth control pill. However, there are patients who have had neither of these hormonal conditions who still get the disease. And even some men occasionally get it, a fact that no one has adequately explained. It must not take much of a disruption of hormones to cause it, however. Some women who took the pill for only a few months, or had a single pregnancy, had pigment form in later years, under the influence of bright sun exposure.

And right there is the key to permanent help for melasma: avoidance of the sun. No woman, regardless of the steps and medicines you'll read about in this chapter, has ever improved permanently without taking major measures to screen herself from the sun and fluorescent light, which we also know will induce this pigment to form.

Melasma is a very difficult condition to treat. Thank goodness we now have superefficient sunscreens, like Solbar PF Ultra 50, which filter out almost all the ultraviolet light, but even with this sunscreen, it's absolutely necessary to wear a good protective layer of cosmetics to protect from the visible light that also induces pigment production.

For years, dermatologists have advised sunlight restriction and topical depigmenters, such as hydroquinone. But not until the formulation of the advanced vehicle used in Neutrogena's Melanex did we have any real success in eliminating melasma. Even then it was a painfully slow process, until investigators discovered that adding Retin-A to the mixture made it extremely effective in removing the excess pigment.

Here's the formula that your dermatologist probably already knows:

Mix one bottle (30cc) Melanex with 7.5cc of Retin-A (0.05%) Solution. Shake well before use. Apply twice daily to pigmented areas.

This combination was found to be physically stable and chemically compatible for six months at room temperature.

Keep in mind, however, that no amount of medication will help this problem without light avoidance. Of course, avoiding light will do a lot more for you than just lighten up your pigment—maybe all women should develop a touch of melasma, just so their dermatologists will recommend that they avoid light for the rest of their lives. *Nothing* could be healthier for skin, as we already know.

If the Retin-A/Melanex mix is applied religiously twice a day for several months, the pigmented areas will gradually start to lighten. But it's a long-term battle, and you may have to stay on the medicine for months to years to prevent a severe recurrence.

Keratosis Pilaris

Are you one of those people who cringe every time you touch the backs of your arms? Those of you with a problem called keratosis pilaris already know exactly what I mean by the term. In my private practice, KP is somewhere in the top 20 most common dermatologic complaints.

This condition is one of many "across-the-room" diagnoses, as my chief of dermatology used to call them. That means that the first-year residents in dermatology are supposed to be able to spot this condition from clear across the examining room, and indeed, many of them can, after a few days' practice in a well-populated skin clinic.

You can always spot KP by the tremendous number of tiny bumps on the backs of the arms, and sometimes on the cheeks (especially in children), and occasionally on the fronts of the thighs. The bumps are not much of a *medical* problem, per se, but they're one of the worst nuisances that one can have, because the backs of the arms are places that are constantly touched, and because patients with KP rarely have the patience to leave the spots alone. They find too late that picking at these spots not only causes temporary sores but also actual *scars*, if the picking continues for any length of time.

What causes KP? Genetics. Somehow, patients with this condition "chose the wrong ancestors" and inherited the tendency to form these spots. The actual spots or bumps on the arms are plugs around hair follicles.

Youth Alert!

One place where KP should be treated actively is on the face, where it can cause scarring if it is severe. If you have a child under 10 with tiny bumps on the face, get that child to the dermatologist!

These little bumps are extraordinarily difficult to treat. But somewhere in the history of Retin-A, the medicine was tried on this condition and found to work wonderfully. Not that it will *cure* the problem—it will not— but it will certainly ameliorate it, causing the bumps to flatten. It takes several weeks for this effect to occur, however, and in the meantime, one can expect to have a lot of dryness of the treated area and some irritation. The irritation, in my experience, is slightly greater in this area of the body than on the face. That's because the backs of the arms have very little natural oiliness, making the dryness somewhat more pronounced.

And for an even greater effect, a new prescription moisturizer has been produced called Lac-Hydrin (Westwood), which contains 12% lactic acid, a compound that loosens the tightly compacted keratin protein plugs that cause this problem. Lac-Hydrin also softens and moisturizes the skin, which is the perfect combination when a patient is using Retin-A. Beware, however, that the lactic acid in Lac-Hydrin can cause stinging in some patients (that's why it's the only prescription moisturizer), so you *must* cautiously *test* a small area before putting the product all over the affected area.

The best way to do this is called a "use test," in which patients apply the substance on a small, 50-cent-piece-size area of skin similar to the skin for which we intend to use it. For KP, this would be the triceps area, on the back of the upper arm. Use it in the same place for several days before attempting to use it all over. Thus, if you *do*, indeed, have any reactions to it, the adverse effects would be confined to a very limited, easily treated area. We often use this technique to test possible allergens in our patients with suspected cosmetic allergies, and it works like a charm.

I always tell patients that the treatment of KP is a step-wise process. Many people will be happy with the result of Lac-Hydrin alone, or just a mild anti-acne soap like SAStid soap (a first-level acne soap that's a little hard to find, but well worth it if you find a druggist who will order it for you), or Clearasil soap, but many more patients want stronger medication to decrease the bumps completely, so that they cannot be felt at all. While it's not possible to *cure* this condition, it is certainly possible to make it seem like it's not there with a combination of the right treatments.

I must add here that many dermatologists have found it helpful to prescribe extra vitamin A for this problem. While I cannot advise doing this without your dermatologist's prescription, I *can* tell you that this approach *has* worked nicely in many of the patients in whom I've tried it. Can you ever stop the extra vitamin A once the rash has cleared? Only time will tell. One thing is for sure—with regular administration, excess vitamin A *does* build up in the body, and cannot be advised without the direct advice and monitoring of your physician.

Foot Calluses

Someone once said that as soon as you realize you have feet, you've got a problem with them. Calluses are one of the most stubborn problems we see in the dermatology office. I have some patients (usually women, for reasons I'll get to in a minute) who are virtually crippled by these painful nuisances.

In order to understand why these tough bumps of dead skin hurt so much, recall that one of the many functions of the skin is to protect the muscles and skeleton below. On the feet that's a particularly difficult function, which often goes awry, resulting in painful calluses on the skin.

Even *normal* people have some areas of callus formation on the feet—by way of protection of the area of the body with the thickest dead layer. The bottoms of the toes, balls of the feet, and heels are commonly thought of as callused, although those common calluses *are* protective.

Athletes often grow calluses in the spots of frictional contact on their skins, like the palms in gymnasts, the bottoms of the feet in runners, and the edges of the feet in figure skaters, who exert great pressure in that area by bending the skate in turns or pressuring the foot into steadiness. But I see the largest number of calluses in my practice in women wearing tight shoes.

If you think about it, it's almost *logical* for modern women to have calluses, because of the pressures of fashion, which dictate that pointed shoes are the style of today. But the human foot has its *own* dictates, and trying to pack five toes into the sharply pointed space that current shoe styles allow is just not healthy for the foot skin and bony architecture. A case in point will demonstrate this.

One of the most common places for a pressure callus to occur on the feet is between the fourth and fifth toes, where the small toe presses upon the larger fourth toe. While this callus is extremely common in women, I have seen only *one* in a man in my career, proving the relationship between tight-fitting, narrow shoes and localized thickening of the foot skin.

Treatment of calluses has included everything from topical dilute acids to paring the lesions just to keep the pain down to a minimum. Often it was necessary to tell a woman that she'd need to return to the office every few months indefinitely to have her lesions retreated. Until Retin-A came along. Now we can use the 0.1% cream applied nightly to the calluses until they thin out, and then use applications one to three nights per week to keep them thinned tolerably. Yes, this can be an indefinite treatment too, but it's something the patient can do for herself to keep the calluses painless.

The only warning here is that a dermatologist must see you and get you started on this treatment, just like starting Retin-A for anything else. This medicine is an acid, after all, and there is always a chance of it irritating skin, even the thick foot skin. Bottom line? Get your dermatologist's *instructions* before using *any* form of Retin-A for *any* purpose.

Stretch Marks

I mention stretch marks after pregnancy here because at least one clinical dermatologist has had good success treating them with Retin-A after delivery. No formal studies have been done on this as yet, but I'm trying it in a few of my patients, and I think it'll bear watching over the next few years. Should you start the Retin-A during your pregnancy on the stretch marks that are actually forming? The company says the drug is not indicated in pregnancy, so that's a decision for you, your dermatologist, and your gynecologist to make as a team. Most will not permit it, and you should not try it by yourself!

There are a host of other conditions in which Retin-A has been tried—some it helped, and some it didn't, and a very few it made worse. But for the most part, they are relatively rare conditions that can be discussed individually with your dermatologist, and for which some other effective therapies do exist. I encourage you to discuss every skin disease with him, since he'll be your final guide. Once again, this book is *not* intended to function as a home medical care book, with a few exceptions, such as the chapter on dry skin, so the absolute best advice I can give you for *any* skin condition is to seek your dermatologist's advice.

INDEX

Books Recommended in *Retin-A and Other Youth Miracles*
(To order, please use the form on the next page)

Cosmetic Surgery for Women by Paula Moynahan, M.D. ... $18.95
Highly recommended by Dr. Bark for those who want to know more about plastic surgery to enhance beauty.

Skin Secrets by Joseph Bark, M.D. $18.95
In this book, Dr. Bark gives many tips on naturally enhancing the skin of every member of the family. Included are sections on: skin infections, acne-scarred skin, skin cancers, moles, and melanomas.

Retin-A and Other Youth Miracles by Joseph Bark, M.D... $17.95

Other Health Titles from Prima Publishing

Good Cholesterol, Bad Cholesterol by Eli M. Roth, M.D. and Sandra Streicher, RN $15.95
Praised by experts as the finest book on cholesterol, this book covers every aspect of the cholesterol equation in a clearly understandable style. "A valuable guide to the benefits of a disease-preventive lifestyle." William C. DeVries, M.D.

Controlling High Blood Pressure edited by Frans H.H. Leenen, M.D. and R. Brian Haynes, M.D................................ $15.95
In this book, 10 of North America's top hypertension specialists, each writing a chapter, cover every aspect of dealing with hypertension. Highly informative, comprehensive, and easy to understand.

Immune for Life by Arnold Fox, M.D. and Barry Fox $17.95
In the final analysis, most diseases are caused by a failure of the immune system to respond correctly. In *Immune for Life*, Dr. Fox shows the reader how to adopt a lifestyle that promotes a strong immune system, which he calls "our doctor within." Included is a program encompassing nutrition, mental attitude, and physical exercise.

Health-Related Cookbooks

Lean and Luscious, and ***More Lean and Luscious*** by Bobbie Hinman and Millie Snyder .... each book $14.95
These two cookbooks each offer over 400 recipes. Each recipe is designed for today's low-fat, low-cholesterol, high-fiber lifestyle. Each recipe comes with at-a-glance nutritional breakdown. Spiral combbound for easy reading.

Dairy-Free Cookbook by Jane Zukin........................ $18.95
For people with little or no milk tolerance, this is a life saver. Included are recipes for both adults and children, and guidelines for eating out. Recommended for gastroenterologists, internists, and all who suffer from milk allergy or lactase deficiency.

FILL IN AND MAIL . . . TODAY

PRIMA PUBLISHING
P.O. BOX 1260RET
ROCKLIN, CA 95677

USE YOUR VISA/MC AND ORDER BY PHONE:
(916) 624-5718 (M–F 9–4 PST)

Dear People at Prima,
I'd like to order the following titles:

Quantity	Title	Amount
_____	_____	_____
_____	_____	_____
_____	_____	_____
_____	_____	_____
_____	_____	_____
	Subtotal	$_____
	Postage & Handling	$ 3.00
	Sales Tax	$_____
	TOTAL (U.S. funds only)	$_____

☐ Check enclosed for $_____ (payable to Prima Publishing)
   Charge my ☐ MasterCard   ☐ Visa

Account No. _____ Exp. Date _____

Signature _____

Your Name _____

Address _____

City/State/Zip _____

Daytime Telephone _____

YOU MUST BE SATISFIED, OR YOUR MONEY BACK !!!
Thank You for Your Order